Neck Dissections

Colour Atlas of Surgical Technique

Neck Dissections
Colour Atlas of Surgical Technique

Jesus E. Medina MD
Professor of Otolaryngology
University of Oklahoma
College of Medicine
Oklahoma City, Oklahoma, USA

Nilesh R. Vasan MD
Associate Professor of Otolaryngology
University of Oklahoma
College of Medicine
Oklahoma City, Oklahoma, USA

Foreword
Robert M. Byers

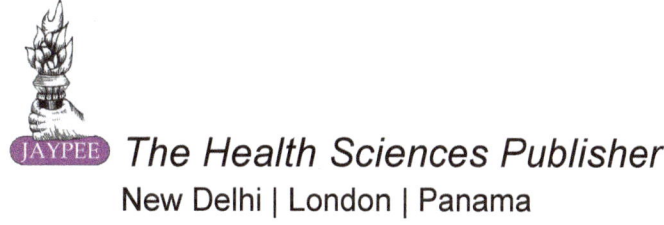

JAYPEE *The Health Sciences Publisher*
New Delhi | London | Panama

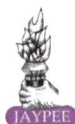 **Jaypee Brothers Medical Publishers (P) Ltd**

Headquarters
Jaypee Brothers Medical Publishers (P) Ltd.
4838/24, Ansari Road, Daryaganj
New Delhi 110 002, India
Phone: +91-11-43574357
Fax: +91-11-43574314
E-mail: jaypee@jaypeebrothers.com

Overseas Offices
J.P. Medical Ltd.
83, Victoria Street, London
SW1H 0HW (UK)
Phone: +44-20 3170 8910
Fax: +44(0)20 3008 6180
E-mail: info@jpmedpub.com

Jaypee Brothers Medical Publishers (P) Ltd.
17/1-B, Babar Road, Block-B, Shaymali
Mohammadpur, Dhaka-1207
Bangladesh
Mobile: +08801912003485
E-mail: jaypeedhaka@gmail.com

Jaypee-Highlights Medical Publishers Inc.
City of Knowledge, Bld. 235, 2nd Floor, Clayton
Panama City, Panama
Phone: +1 507-301-0496
Fax: +1 507-301-0499
E-mail: cservice@jphmedical.com

Jaypee Brothers Medical Publishers (P) Ltd.
Bhotahity, Kathmandu, Nepal
Phone: +977-9741283608
E-mail: kathmandu@jaypeebrothers.com

Website: www.jaypeebrothers.com
Website: www.jaypeedigital.com

© 2018, Jaypee Brothers Medical Publishers

Inquiries for bulk sales may be solicited at: jaypee@jaypeebrothers.com

Neck Dissections: Colour Atlas of Surgical Technique

First Edition: **2018**

ISBN 978-93-86322-28-9

Printed at

Dedicated to

Robert M. Byers MD

Extraordinary head and neck surgeon and teacher,
a trusted mentor and a loyal friend.

His contributions are part of the foundation for the current management
of the neck in patients with cancer of the head and neck.

Jesus E. Medina MD

Dedicated to

My preceptor and friend Jesus E. Medina whose wisdom, enthusiasm, attention to detail and selflessness have helped me and countless others master neck dissection.

Nilesh R. Vasan MD

Foreword

In surgery art has a real need because depending on the finesse and perfection of its artistry,
the success of a surgical procedure largely and sometimes entirely depends.
It is the art of the sculpturer rendered with heroism and the skill of a life-saver.
William D Haggard (1872-1940)

It is July 1980. The weather in Houston, Texas is typical of its summers—hot and humid. A group of aspiring young hopeful doctors have gathered to start their fellowships in head and neck surgery at MD Anderson Cancer Center. One of these young men is destined to become a world class head and neck cancer surgeon. Today, we all know him and admire him as Jesus E Medina.

Dr Medina is a man who has devoted his entire professional life to the compassionate care of patients with head and neck cancer. He has worked hard to hone his surgical skills, expand his understanding of its causes and has developed and refined various surgical procedures in its treatment. Every patient with head and neck cancer has profoundly benefitted.

My involvement with Jesus began during his initial interview and continued throughout his fellowship and his years as a faculty member in the Department of Head and Neck Surgery at MD Anderson. Later when he moved to Oklahoma and became Chairman of the Department of Otolaryngology—Head and Neck Surgery at the University of Oklahoma we continued our association. I have enjoyed my multiple roles guiding his surgery during the formative years and mentoring him as he progressed in his academic career. We frequently shared the roles of teaching medical students, surgical residents and fellows and practicing colleagues in the United States and around the world. We were part of panels, symposiums, and in writing articles in books and journals. What was especially gratifying to me was when two of my sons decided to pursue a career in Otolaryngology—Head and Neck Surgery. Dr Medina trained both of them in his Department at Oklahoma. Both today are very respected and successful in private practice.

Before critiquing *Neck Dissections: Colour Atlas of Surgical Technique*, I believe it is appropriate to provide a brief historical perspective of neck dissections in general. Anyone who discusses, writes or teaches about the care of patients with head and neck cancer must address the treatment of the neck. In the past, if the cancer had spread to the neck, the patient was considered either not a candidate for surgery or incurable. Gradually overtime, surgeons became more aggressive in their conceptual approach to the neck treatment. Better anesthesia, safe and available blood replacement, appropriate use of antibiotics and fine-tuning their technical skills facilitated this advancement.

In 1961, Dr Hayes Martin, a prominent surgeon, working in Memorial Hospital, New York City published a paper describing a type of neck dissection which removed the nodes in the neck from the jaw bone to the clavicle. The sternocleidomastoid (SCM) muscle, the internal jugular vein and the spinal accessory nerve were included with the nodes. This "groundbreaking" procedure became known as the radical neck dissection. Its use became so ingrained in the lexicon of head and neck surgeons that any suggestion of a lesser procedure was considered surgical heresy. It took considerable patience, determination and even academic courage for young surgeons from the United States, Spain and Brazil to explore and study the data from the use of other possible operational arrows to put in the quiver of neck dissection treatment. With the use of better radiologic studies of the neck and a more thorough pathologic evaluation of the neck contents following a completion of the operation, less radical operations were proposed. The new procedures were not only appropriate for removing obviously cancerous nodes but also were effective in removing nodes not clinically involved but potentially containing subclinical cancer. All major anatomic structures of esthetic and functional significance could be preserved. As a result, the patient today can be offered surgical options which are oncologically sound with less morbidity and better tailored to the site of origin of the cancer and its extent in the neck.

Neck Dissections: Colour Atlas of Surgical Technique is a significant work, guaranteed to take a place in the top tier of all such surgical guides. When you see the table of contents you immediately grasp the scope and breath of this book. All of the various types of neck dissections are readily recognized. Even some are described which are not always included in similar publications. The classification of the dissection is updated and several useful incisions are illustrated and described. The text is well organized and focused. Using very precise language, each of the procedures are developed step by step along with helpful technical maneuvers that can expose and preserve vital anatomic structures. The photography of the actual dissections performed by Dr Medina in the operating room is spectacular. The accurate artistic representations are coupled with these real operations. This coupling of the visual with the written is very useful in enhancing the reader's comprehension of each procedure. These complex dissections are beautifully revealed by the painter's brush while Jesus Medina magically defines them with his scalpel. It is obvious that the operating room is his studio. I have always believed that surgery, in its purest, is an art form. Jesus is an artist no different really from a sculptor. I am so pleased that he has decided to publish this book. It will continue to be an educational requirement for any surgeon who cares for the head and neck cancer patient and who performs the indicated neck dissections.

In 2015, Dr Medina semi-retired. He continues to be active teaching eager learners and contributing to the literature. He will always be a caring father of his 3 children and a devoted husband to his wife Libby. We continue to remain close friends.

Robert M. Byers MD
Former Alando J Ballantyne Professor of Surgery
Department of Head and Neck Surgery
at MD Anderson Tumor Institute
Houston, Texas, USA

Preface

The impetus to put together this Atlas has grown over several decades. For over 30 years, I have had the privilege of teaching about neck dissection to residents and fellows, and of speaking to audiences around the world on this topic. In these presentations I have often relied on intraoperative photographs and drawings to describe different aspects of surgical technique of one or more neck dissections. Invariably an audience member or student would inquire about the availability of a source describing and illustrating the techniques as I had presented them. Time and time again, I had to admit that such a source did not exist.

Additionally, I have been privileged to author chapters on neck dissection for many of the existing atlases and textbooks of Otolaryngology and Head and Neck Surgery. However, the constraints of "space" dedicated to these chapters limited the details that could be included, and reduced the description of technique to a "broad-stroke" rather than a finely nuanced presentation. In addition, the illustrations that accompanied these publications were often limited to black and white line drawings or colour cartoons.

Consequently, for many years now, I have entertained the idea of compiling an atlas that would be devoted exclusively to neck dissections. I envisioned a work that would present a properly comprehensive, detailed description of each operation, divided in practical steps based upon how we teach these operations to our trainees. It would include, side-by-side with the corresponding text, unique, colour, life-like artist renditions of the different surgical maneuvers and anatomic structures, pertinent to each step of the operation.

As luck, or fate, would have it, while making rounds one evening about 15 years ago, I happened upon a pharmaceutical advertising poster that depicted a drawing of the musculature and vessels of the neck. I was struck by the realism of its colours and proportions. Immediately, I embarked on a search for the creator of such an impressive drawing, and several days later, I discovered the gifted, Swedish-born illustrator, Ms. Lena Lyons. I contacted her by phone about the idea of drawing to illustrate surgical procedures. Fortunately, she lived in Ventura, CA, and we subsequently met for several hours at Los Angeles International Airport. She shared my enthusiasm for the project, and eagerly embarked on our shared endeavor, spending countless hours in the operating room, observing us perform the different types of neck dissections, sketching, patiently adjusting her sketches and finally producing the realistic drawings of extraordinary quality, accuracy and beauty that illustrate this Atlas. Unfortunately, Lena passed away a few years ago. I regret that she is not able to see the final product that she was so instrumental in creating. Lena Lyons was not only a gifted artist—she was an exceptional human being whose work ethic and friendship have been an inspiration to me.

Anyone who has written a book knows the many hours of work it requires, the preoccupation that makes one almost absent minded to anything else, especially when assembling the "final" version of it. None of the work for this Atlas would have been possible for me without the understanding and loving support of my dear wife, Libby. Therefore I consider this coveted accomplishment not so much mine but ours. As such, both of us felt it would be fitting to dedicate the book to Robert Byers, MD our dear friend and my mentor. In addition to his contributions to the literature in the area of neck dissection as the former Alando J Ballantyne Professor of Surgery at the MD Anderson Tumor Institute, Robert Byers personifies, in my view, the ideal surgeon: knowledgeable, caring and technically masterful.

The Atlas is divided in chapters that each address one type of neck dissection, beginning with a brief account of how the operation came to be, the indications for it and then a detailed description of the surgical technique.

When appropriate, we have supplemented the colour drawings with black and white line drawings and intraoperative photographs.

This Atlas is part of a work in progress. In the near future, the surgical steps described here and now illustrated with drawings will be supplemented with clear, high-definition video segments. Furthermore, as robotic surgery matures and becomes more common place, similar descriptions of robot-assisted neck dissection will be included. My friend, colleague and co-author Nilesh Vasan is carrying the baton in our race towards that end.

It is our hope that anyone interested in head and neck oncologic surgery, trainees and practitioners alike, will find the descriptions in this Atlas useful to either learn or to refresh their memory about the surgical technique of the different neck dissections.

Jesus E. Medina MD

Acknowledgments

I wish to honor the memory of Lena Lyons whose untimely death has deprived us of an outstanding artist and my friend. Her wonderful illustrations are a pillar of this Atlas.

Jesus E. Medina

Contents

CHAPTER 1

Classification of Neck Dissections

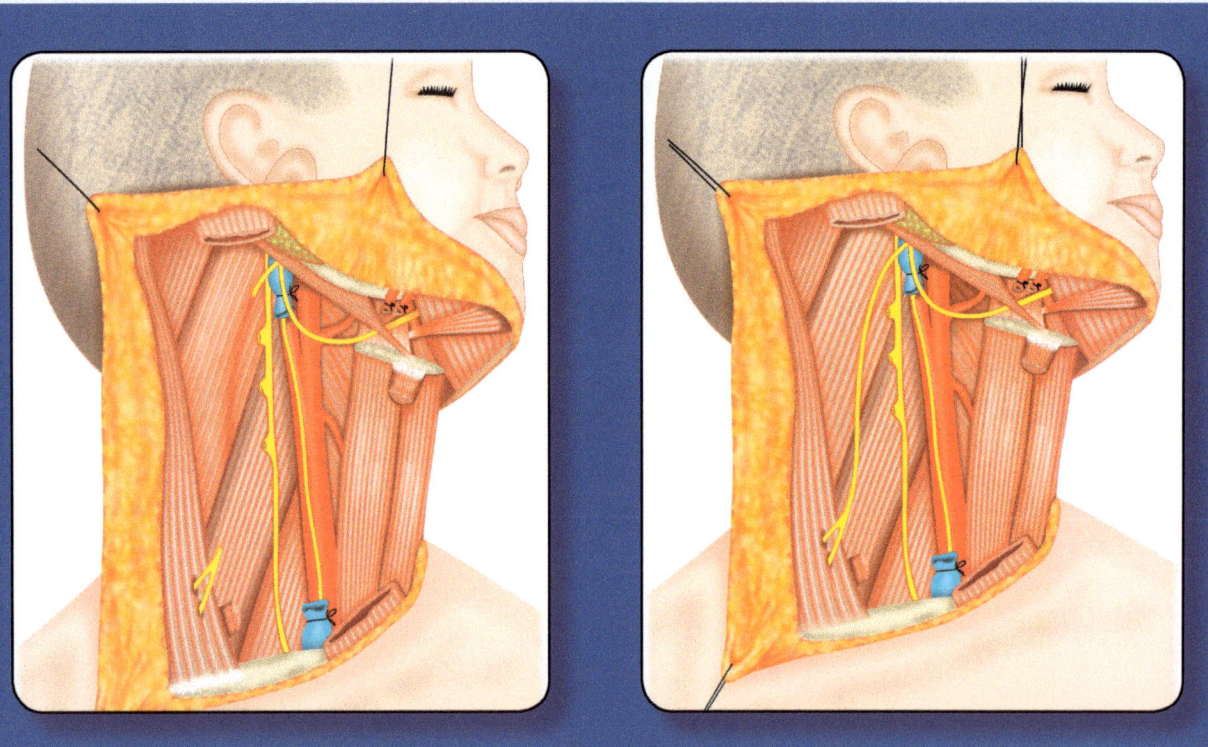

INTRODUCTION

Several cervical lymph node dissections are currently used for the surgical treatment of the neck in patients with cancer of the head and neck region. A standardized nomenclature to refer to these operations is based on a common nomenclature for the groups of lymph nodes in the neck. A time-honored system that uses Roman numerals to designate the groups of lymph node in different regions of the neck is almost universally applicable. In this system, six levels (I–VI) are used that encompass the complete topographic anatomy of the neck. In addition, sublevels have been introduced into some levels to designate zones that may have clinical significance[1] (Fig. 1). Level VII is added to designate the upper mediastinal nodes.

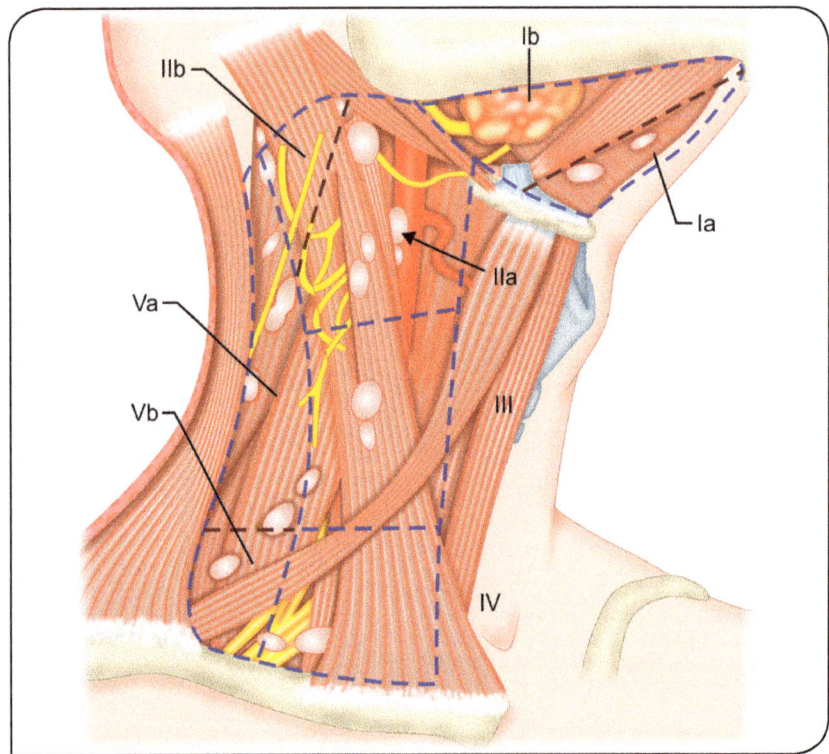

Fig. 1: Lymph node groups or levels of the neck.

LEVEL I

Level I is divided into two sublevels which are as follows:
1. *Sublevel IA (Submental)*: It includes the lymph nodes within the inferiorly based triangle bound by the anterior belly of the digastric muscles and the hyoid bone.
2. *Sublevel IB (Submandibular)*: It includes the lymph nodes within the boundaries of the anterior belly of the digastric muscle, the stylohyoid muscle and the inferior border of the body of the mandible.

LEVEL II

Level II (upper jugular or jugulodigastric): It includes the lymph nodes located around the upper third of the internal jugular vein (IJV) and adjacent to the cephalic portion of the spinal accessory nerve (XIN), extending from the level of the skull base to the level of the inferior border of the hyoid. The anterior or medial boundary is the stylohyoid muscle (the radiological correlate is the vertical plane defined by the posterior surface of the submandibular gland) and the posterior (lateral) boundary is the posterior border of the sternocleidomastoid muscle (SCMM). Two sublevels are recognized in level II, which are as follows:
1. *Sublevel IIA*: It includes the nodes located anterior and medial to the vertical plane defined by the XIN.
2. *Sublevel IIB*: It includes the nodes located posterior and superior to the vertical plane defined by the XIN.

LEVEL III

Level III (midjugular or jugulo-omohyoid): It designates the lymph nodes located around the middle third of the IJV extending from the inferior border of the hyoid bone to the inferior border of the cricoid cartilage. The anterior or medial boundary is the lateral border of the sternohyoid muscle, and the posterior or lateral boundary is the posterior border of the SCMM.

LEVEL IV

Level IV (lower jugular): It encompasses the lymph nodes located around the lower third of the IJV extending from the inferior border of the cricoid cartilage to the clavicle.

The anatomic boundary that separates the medial border of levels III and IV from the lateral border of level VI traditionally has been the lateral border of the sternohyoid muscle, a landmark that cannot be easily discerned on imaging studies. Therefore, the medial aspect of the common carotid artery has been suggested as an alternate boundary to separate these levels in an axial plane in imaging studies.

LEVEL V

Level V (posterior triangle): It comprises predominantly the lymph nodes located along the inferior portions of the XIN and the transverse cervical artery. The supraclavicular nodes are also included in level V. The superior boundary is the apex formed by convergence of the sternocleidomastoid and trapezius muscles. The inferior boundary is the clavicle, the anterior boundary is the posterior border of the SCMM and the posterior boundary is the anterior border of the trapezius muscle. A horizontal plane marking the inferior border of the anterior cricoid arch separates two sublevels, which are as follows:
1. *Sublevel VA*: It includes the nodes located above the plane of the inferior border of the cricoid, which are most of the nodes around the spinal accessory nerve.
2. *Sublevel VB*: It includes the nodes below the cricoid plane, which are the nodes that follow the transverse cervical vessels and the supraclavicular nodes, with the exception of Virchow's node, which is located in level IV.

LEVEL VI

Level VI (anterior or central compartment): Lymph nodes in this level include the pre- and paratracheal nodes, precricoid (Delphian) node and the perithyroidal nodes including the lymph nodes along the recurrent laryngeal nerves. The superior boundary is the hyoid bone, the inferior boundary is the suprasternal notch, and the lateral boundaries are the common carotid arteries.

LEVEL VII

It includes the paratracheal nodes located between the suprasternal notch (the dividing line between levels VI and VII) and the innominate artery.

OTHER LYMPH NODE GROUPS

Lymph nodes in regions not located within these levels should be referred to by the name of their specific nodal group; examples of these are the superior mediastinal, the retropharyngeal, the periparotid, the buccinator, the postauricular and the suboccipital lymph nodes.

RETROPHARYNGEAL LYMPH NODES

Retropharyngeal lymph nodes (RPLNs) are lymph nodes that lie within a pad of adipose tissue located behind the lateral portion of the posterior wall of the pharynx, anterior to the prevertebral fascia and the cervical sympathetic trunk and ganglion, and medial to the internal carotid artery. This pad of adipose tissue extends from about the level of the carotid bifurcation to just below the skull base. The RPLNs are divided into medial and lateral groups; the medial group of nodes lies behind the pharyngeal midline at a level between the first and fourth cervical vertebrae. The lateral group of nodes, better known as the nodes of Rouviere, are contained within a sliver of adipose tissue located immediately medial to the internal carotid artery. The RPLNs receive lymphatic drainage from the nasopharynx, tonsil fossa, the walls of the oropharynx and the hypopharynx, and the posterior ethmoid sinuses.

CLASSIFICATIONS OF NECK DISSECTIONS

The current classification of neck dissections recommended by the American Academy of Otolaryngology—Head and Neck Surgery and the American Head and Neck Society[1] (Table 1) takes into account the groups of lymph nodes of the neck that are removed and secondarily the anatomic structures that are preserved, such as the XIN and the IJV. Because of its simplicity and worldwide acceptance at this time, this classification will be used to designate the neck dissections described in this atlas. Analyzing neck dissections from these two points of view, there are essentially four anatomic types of neck dissections which are as follows:

Table 1: Classifications of neck dissections.

AAOHNS/ASHNS 2001 classification	*2010 proposed classification*

1. Radical neck dissection
2. Modified radical neck dissection
3. Selective neck dissection:
  • SND (I–III/IV)
  • SND (II–IV)
  SND (II–V, postauricular, suboccipital)
  • SND (Level VI)
4. Extended neck dissection
	1. ND (I–V, SCM, IJV, CN XI)
	2. ND (I–V, SCM, IJV)
	  • ND (I–V, IJV, CN XI)
	  • ND (ND I-V, CN XI)
	3. ND (I, II, III/IV)
	  • ND (II, III, IV)
	  • ND (II, III, IV, V, postauricular, suboccipital)
	  • ND (VI)
	4. ND (Levels removed, additional nodes or structures removed)

(AAOHNS: American Academy of Otolaryngology—Head and Neck Surgery; ASHNS: American Society for Head and Neck Surgery; CN XI: Cranial nerve 11; IJV: Internal jugular vein; ND: Neck dissection; SCM: Sternocleidomastoid; SND: Selective neck dissection).

1. *Radical neck dissection (RND)*: In the RND, the lymph node levels I through V are removed along with the SCMM, the IJV, and the XIN (Fig. 2).

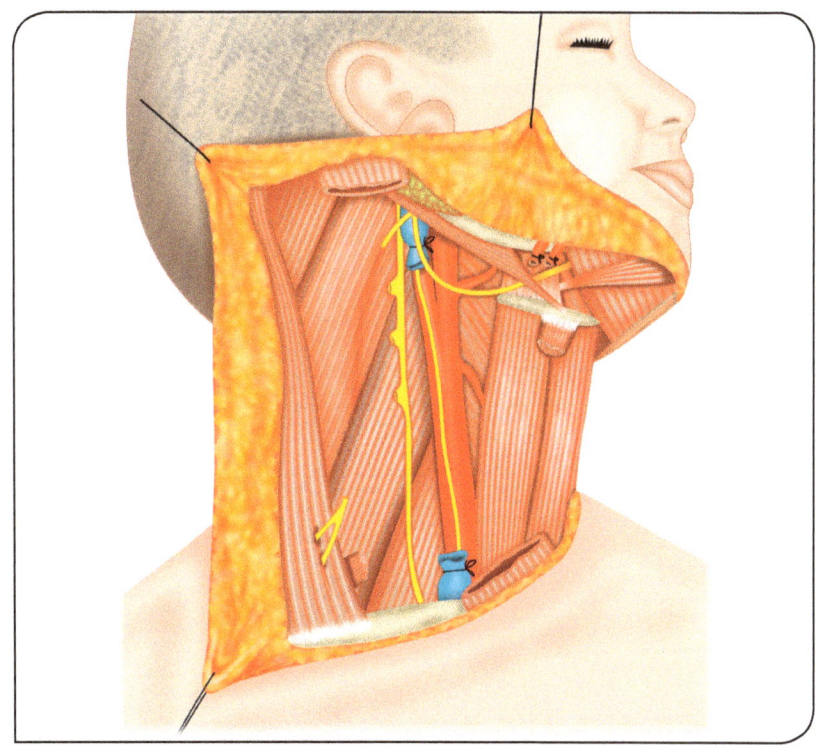

Fig. 2: Radical neck dissection (ND I -V, SCM, IJV, XIN).

2. *Modified radical neck dissections (MRNDs)*: In this type of neck dissection, lymph node levels I through V are removed, as in the RND. However, one or more of the following structures are preserved: SCMM, IJV or the XIN (Figs. 3 and 4).

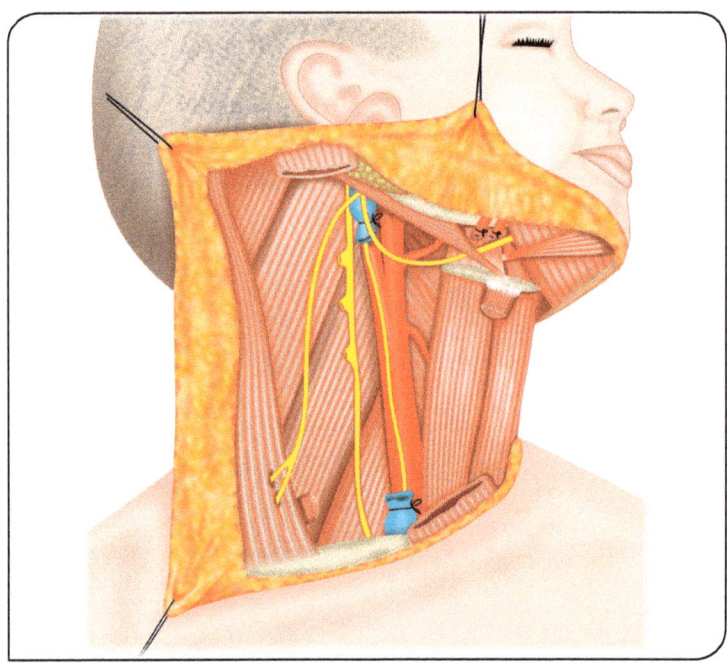

Fig. 3: Modified radical neck dissection (ND) with preservation of the spinal accessory nerve [neck dissection (ND I–V, SCMM, IJV)].

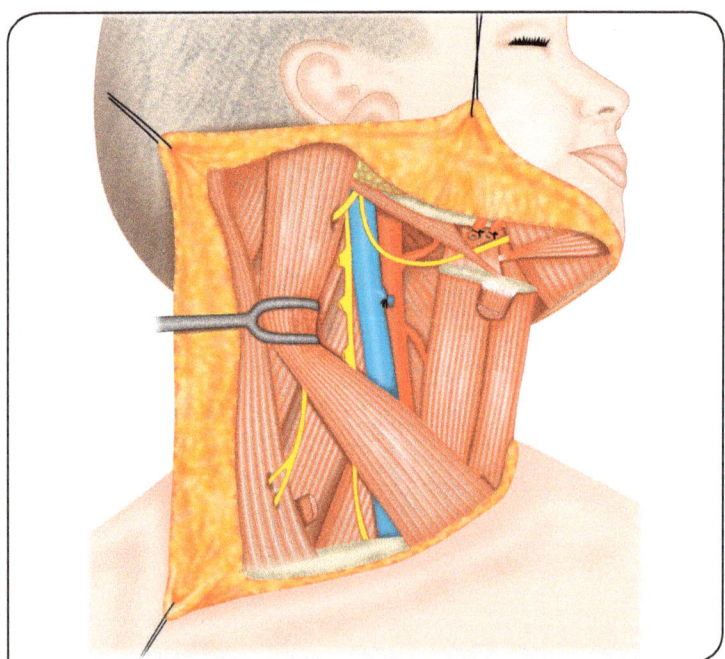

Fig. 4: Modified radical neck dissection (ND) with preservation of the spinal accessory nerve, the internal jugular vein (IJV), and the sternocleidomastoid muscle (SCMM) [ND I–V].

Some clinicians refer to the RND and MRND as "comprehensive" neck dissections, since all five levels of the neck are removed.[2]

3. *Selective neck dissections (SNDs)*: These neck dissections remove selected lymph nodes, based on their risk of containing metastases, which depends upon the location of the primary tumor. The SCMM, IJV and XIN are usually preserved. Four different neck dissections are included in this category, which are as follows:

    (*i*) *Selective neck dissection of levels I–III ("supraomohyoid" neck dissection) and SND of levels I–IV (also referred to as "extended supraomohyoid" neck dissection)*: The lymph nodes removed are those contained in the levels I, II and III. These are the neck dissections commonly used in the treatment of patients with squamous cell carcinoma of the oral cavity (Fig. 5).

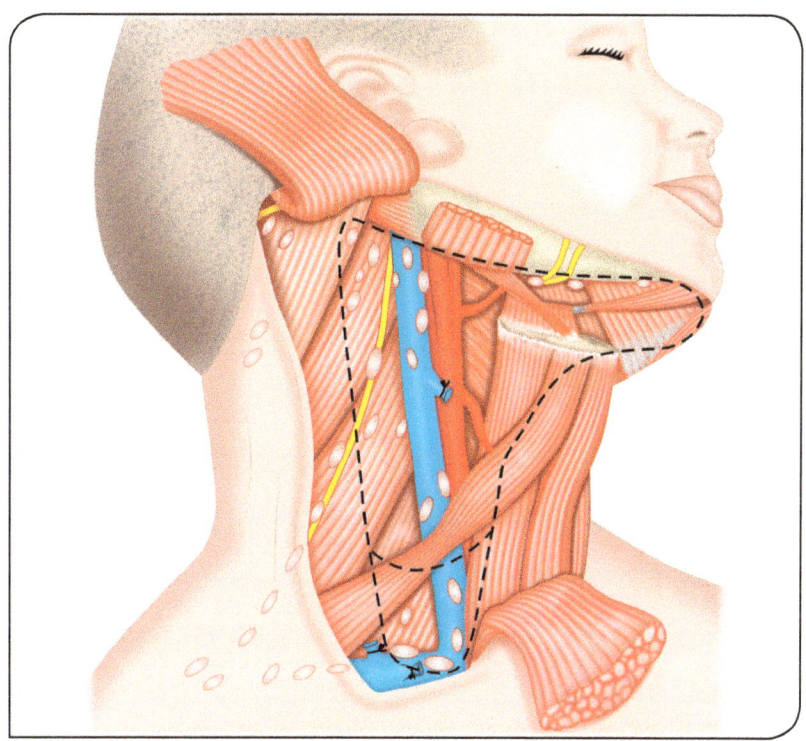

Fig. 5: Selective neck dissection of levels I–III or IV (ND I, II, III or IV).

    (*ii*) *Selective neck dissection of levels II–IV (lateral neck dissection)*: This neck dissection consists of the removal of the lymph nodes in levels II, III and IV. It is commonly used in the treatment of patients with squamous cell carcinoma (SCCA) of the larynx, oropharynx and hypopharynx (Fig. 6).

    (*iii*) *Selective neck dissection of levels II–V, retroauricular and suboccipital nodes (posterolateral neck dissection)*: This operation is done for skin cancers, particularly melanomas, which originate in the posterior-lateral aspect of the scalp and the skin of the neck (Fig. 7).

    (*iv*) *Selective neck dissection of level VI*: This operation, also called "anterior" neck dissection or "central compartment" dissection, consists of the removal of the prelaryngeal, pretracheal and paratracheal lymph nodes. Depending upon the clinical situation, it may be done on one or both sides. It is used in the treatment of patients with cancer of the midline structures of the anterior-inferior aspect of the neck and thoracic inlet, such as the thyroid, the glottic and subglottic regions of the larynx, the pyriform sinus, the cervical esophagus, and trachea.

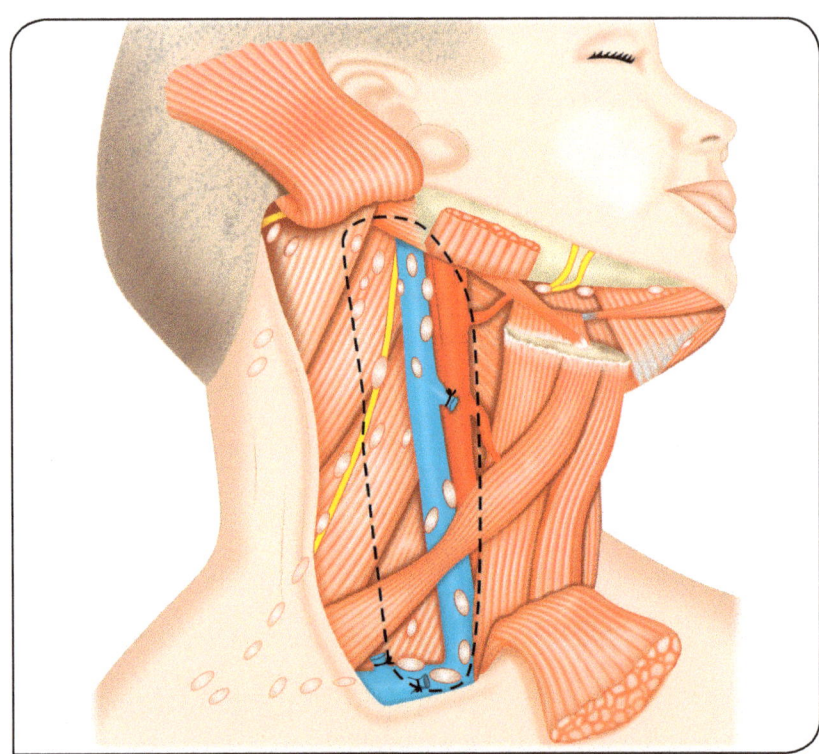

Fig. 6: Selective neck dissection of levels II–IV (ND II, III, IV).

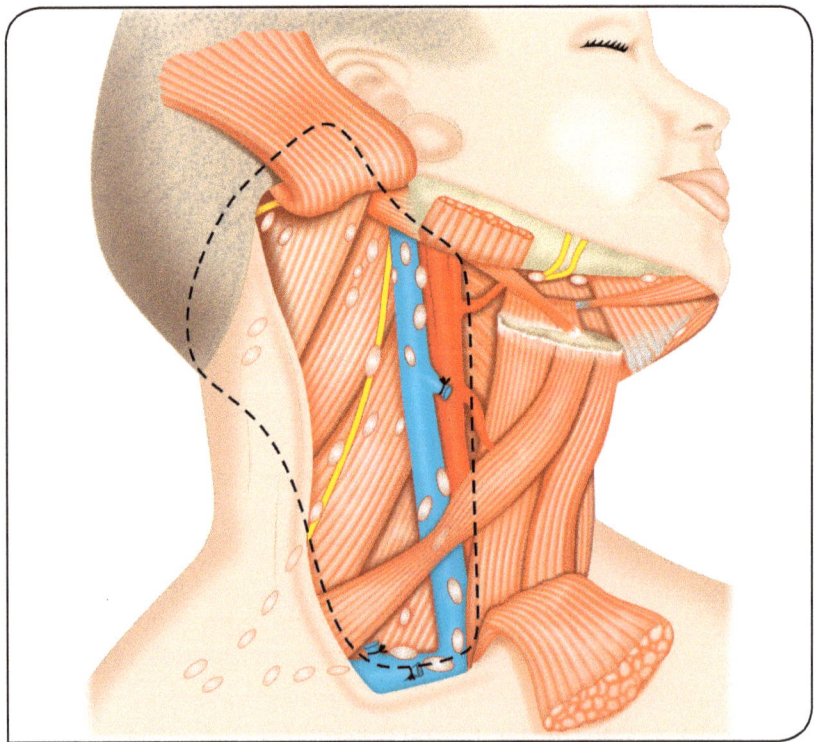

Fig. 7: Posterolateral neck dissection (ND II, III, IV, V, postauricular, and suboccipital).

4. *Extended neck dissection*: This designation is used to indicate that the neck dissection includes either nodal groups (such as the retropharyngeal or superior mediastinal) or nonlymphatic structures (such as skin of the neck, levator scapulae muscle, hypoglossal nerve and carotid artery), which are not ordinarily removed in the other neck dissections.

Other Classifications

Recently, clinicians from around the world have proposed a nomenclature for neck dissections which, if recognized internationally, would be "logical, unambiguous, precise, and easy to remember".[3]

In this classification, the following three descriptors are used to label a neck dissection:

1. "ND" to represent neck dissection which is prefaced by either "L" or "R" for side. If bilateral, each side must be classified independently.
2. The levels and sublevels of lymph nodes removed designated by Roman numerals I through VI in ascending order. For levels that contain sublevels (I, II and V), listing of the level without a sublevel indicates that the entire level (both A and B) was excised.
3. The nonlymphatic structures removed designated by their internationally recognized initials, i.e. SCMM for sternocleidomastoid muscle, IJV for internal jugular vein, and XIN for the spinal accessory nerve.

The potential advantage of this classification is that it conveys precisely the groups of lymph nodes included as well as the nonlymphatic structures removed in a neck dissection. This will allow a standardized reporting and meaningful comparison of outcomes. However, it remains to be seen if it will be adopted widely.

Irrespective of the nomenclature used, it is the responsibility of the surgeon to divide or otherwise orient the neck dissection specimen, identifying the different groups of lymph nodes that it contains immediately after surgery. Only then the pathologist can be expected to render a report that is useful clinically and prognostically. Such a report describes the location and number of lymph nodes examined, the number of nodes that contain cancer, and the presence or absence of capsular extension of tumor.

REFERENCES

1. Robbins KT, Shaha AR, Medina JE, et al. Consensus statement on the classification and terminology of neck dissection. Arch Otolaryngol Head Neck Surg. 2008;134(5):536-8.
2. Medina JE. A rational classification of neck dissections. Otolaryngol Head Neck Surg. 1989;100(3):169-76.
3. Ferlito A, Robbins KT, Shah JP, et al. Proposal for a rational classification of neck dissections. Head Neck. 2011;33(3):445-50.

CHAPTER 2

Incisions

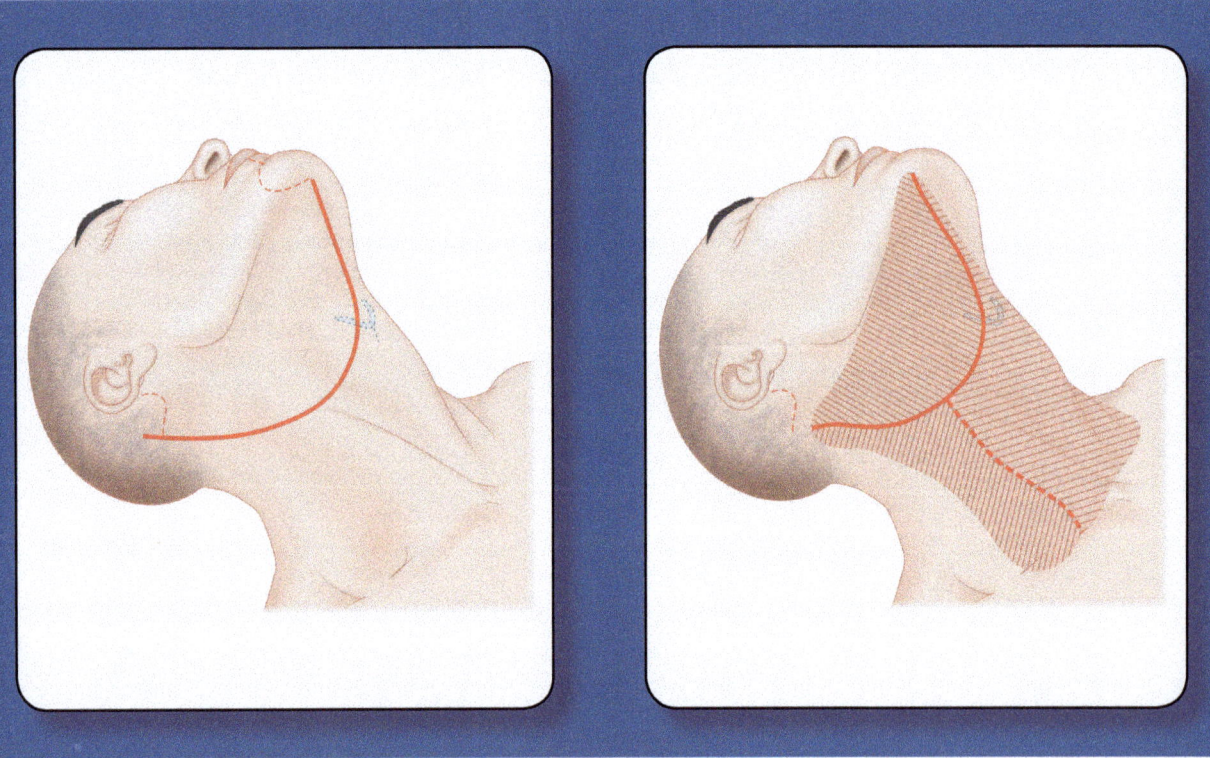

SELECTION OF THE INCISION

The choice of incision in the neck is critical in the preoperative planning of surgery for tumors of the head and neck. The ideal incision allows adequate exposure of all the lymph node levels that need to be dissected, as well as easy access to and ample exposure of the primary tumor. In addition, it should not compromise potential reconstructive options. Preferably, the incision avoids trifurcations, especially if the trifurcation is located over or near the carotid artery. Such trifurcate incisions can be complicated by necrosis of the tips of the skin flaps, particularly in the previously radiated patient. When this occurs, it may result in exposure of the carotid artery, which requires prompt attention to cover the artery and repair the skin defect with nonirradiated skin, muscle or both.

Fortunately, today, there are several practical incisions that the head and neck surgeon can choose, depending on the following factors:

- *Location of the primary tumor*: The ideal incision to perform a neck dissection for a squamous cell carcinoma of the oral cavity would be different than the incision ideal when the primary tumor is in the larynx or hypopharynx.
- *Stage of the neck*: The incision that is ideal to perform an elective neck dissection, which is limited to certain lymph node groups, may be different than that necessary to perform a therapeutic neck dissection, particularly when lymph nodes in several levels of the neck are involved by metastases.
- *Type of cancer*: The ideal incision would be different when a neck dissection is performed in conjunction with a thyroidectomy for medullary thyroid cancer than that which is ideal in a case of melanoma of the skin of the neck.
- *Previous performance of an ill-planned excisional or incisional biopsy of a neck node*: In such cases, it is advisable to excise the biopsy scar, preferably in continuity with the neck dissection specimen. Needless to say that this will influence the type of incision to be used for the neck dissection.

In this chapter, we describe those incisions that we have found practical and have used many times, over the years, to perform the entire gamut of neck dissections.

MODIFIED SCHOBINGER INCISION (FIG. 1)

This incision is suitable to perform a dissection of levels I–V; it can be extended easily into a lip-splitting incision to excise a tumor of the oral cavity or oropharynx. It can also be extended into the chest, creating a robust skin flap that can be rotated upwards to repair a defect resulting from removing the skin overlying the mandible or from removing the skin of the lower cheek. It can also be used to repair the defect resulting from excising a "lymph node biopsy" scar in the submandibular area.

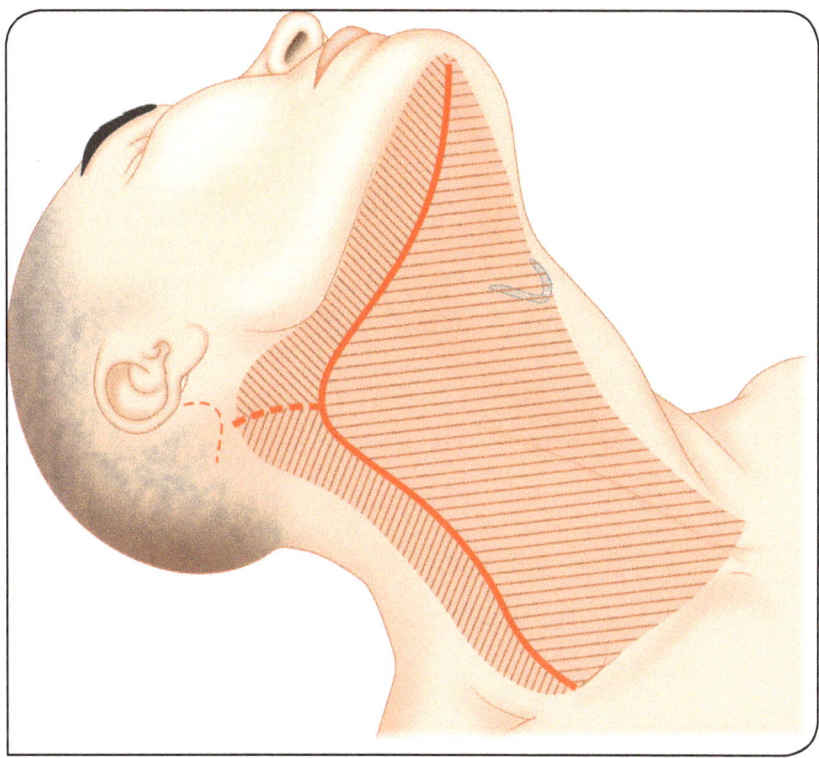

Fig. 1: Modified Schobinger incision. The areas of the neck easily accessible with this incision are shaded.

MODIFIED MCFEE INCISION (FIG. 2)

The McFee incision can be modified by making the superior incision curved upwards on both ends, as opposed to a straight line. It is suitable to perform a neck dissection of levels I–V. It can also be extended anteriorly to split the lip to approach the oral cavity or the oropharynx. It is particularly useful to do a neck dissection in conjunction with a thyroidectomy, when there are palpable metastases in level I and other levels of the neck.

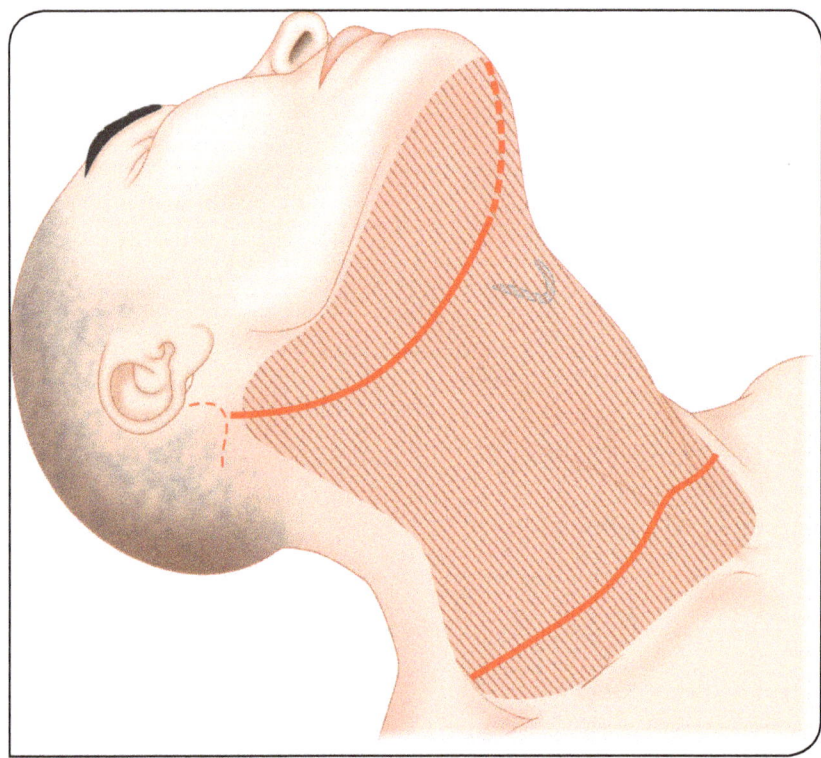

Fig. 2: Modified McFee incision. The areas of the neck easily accessible with these incisions are shaded.

MODIFIED MCFEE INCISION (FIGS. 3A TO C)

A. The McFee incision can also be modified by making the superior incision short and placing it in a natural crease of the neck at about the level of the hyoid bone. We find this incision to be particularly useful in children and young women that need a neck dissection in conjunction with a thyroidectomy, when there are palpable metastases in level V and in levels II, III or IV.

B. Intraoperative photograph showing a thyroidectomy done in conjunction with a modified radical neck dissection (levels II–V, preserving the internal jugular vein (IJV), sternocleidomastoid muscles (SCMM) and spinal accessory nerve (XIN).

C. Postoperative photograph showing the cosmetic results.

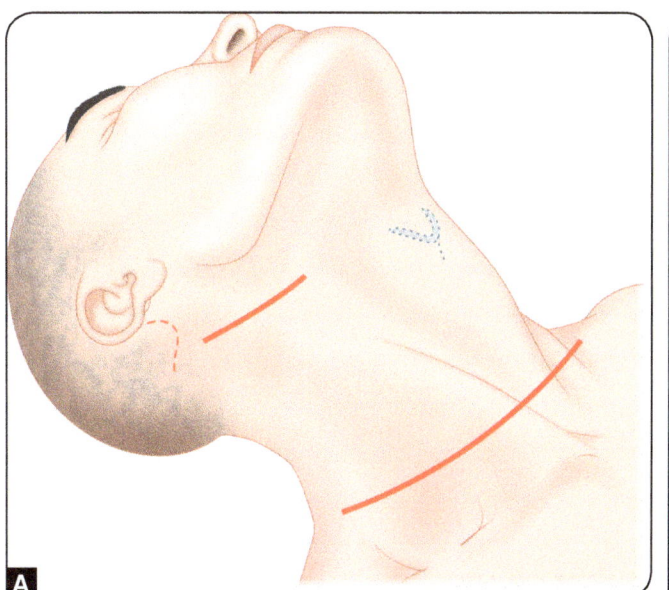
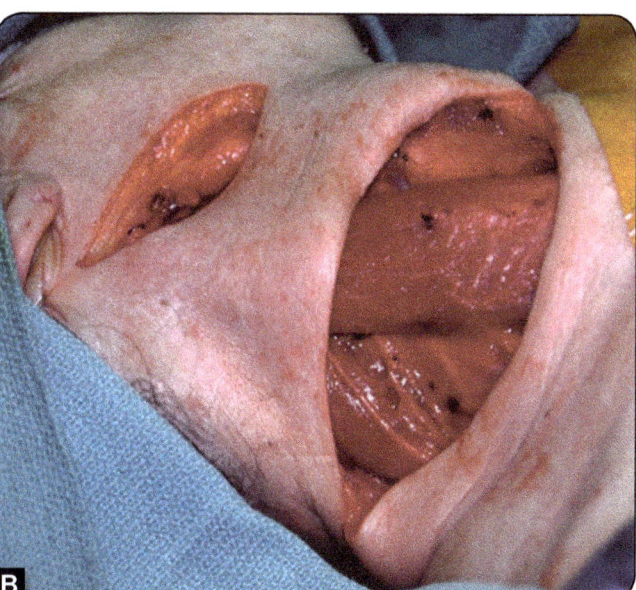
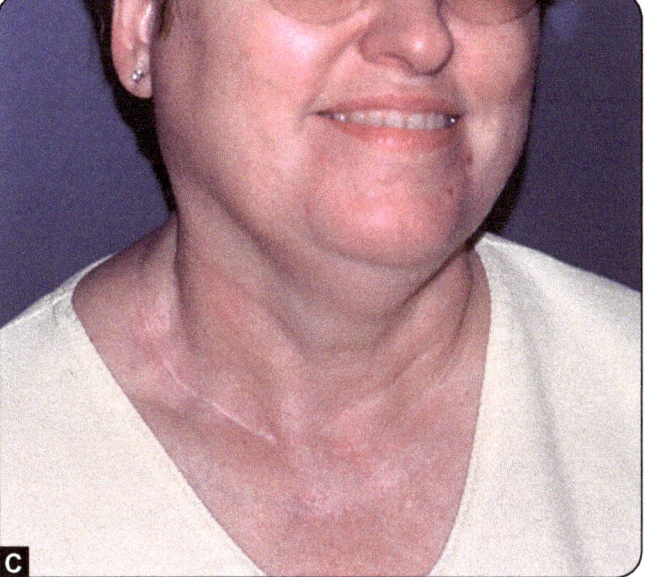

Figs. 3A to C: Modified McFee incision; postoperative appearance.

UNILATERAL APRON-LIKE INCISION (FIG. 4A)

This incision is particularly useful to perform a selective neck dissection of levels I–III, especially when the surgeon anticipates having to split the lip to approach the primary tumor. If, in the course of the operation, it becomes necessary to extend the dissection to level IV or level V, and the exposure is limited, a descending limb can be added. In such cases, we prefer to place the descending limb at about the level of the external jugular vein (Fig. 4B). Placing it further posteriorly may jeopardize the blood supply to the tip of the anterior inferior flap.

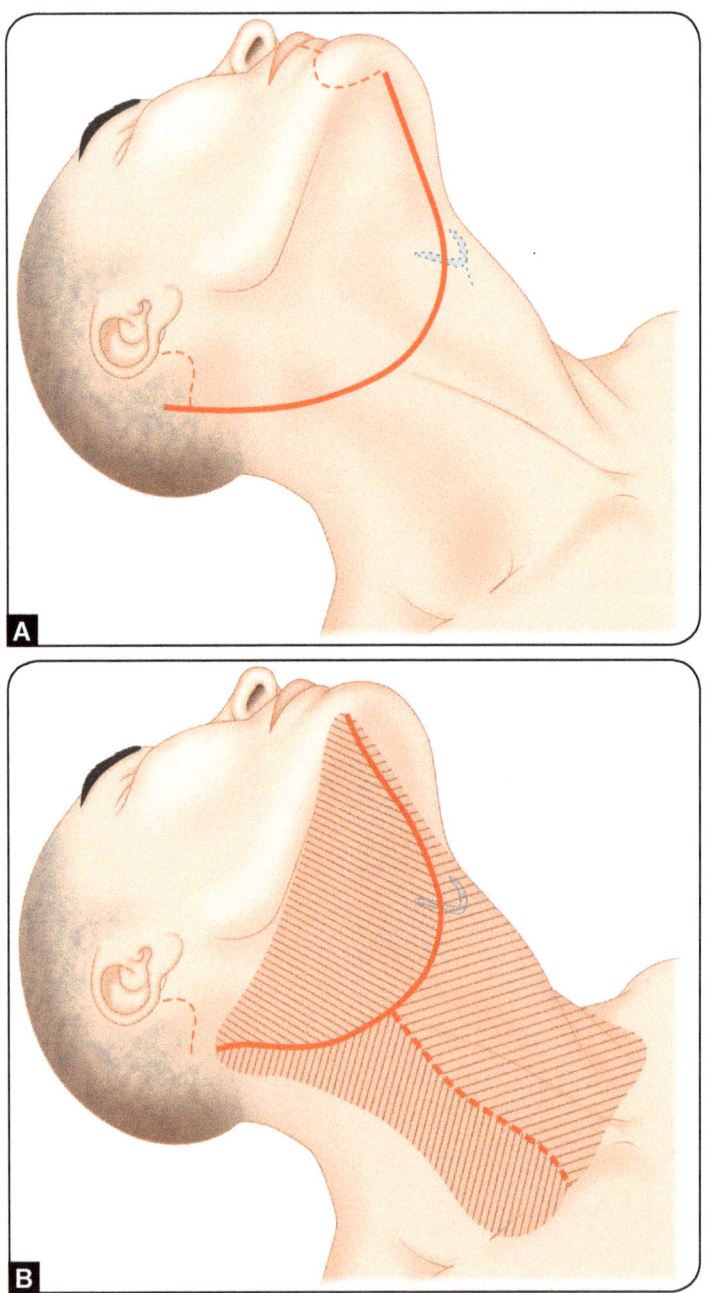

Figs. 4A and B: Unilateral apron-like incision. Areas of the neck easily accessible with this incision.

UPPER TRANSVERSE INCISION (FIGS. 5A TO D)

A. This incision extends from the mid or posterior third of the SCMM posteriorly to the midline anteriorly. It is placed in a natural crease in the upper lateral aspect of the neck at about the level of the thyrohyoid membrane.
B. If needed for additional exposure, the posterior end can be extended upwards towards the area behind the mastoid tip; anteriorly, it can be extended beyond the midline to provide additional exposure to dissect the submental triangle or upwards into a lip-splitting incision.
C. Intraoperative photograph showing an upper transverse incision.
D. Intraoperative photograph showing the ample exposure to complete a selective neck dissection of levels I–III.

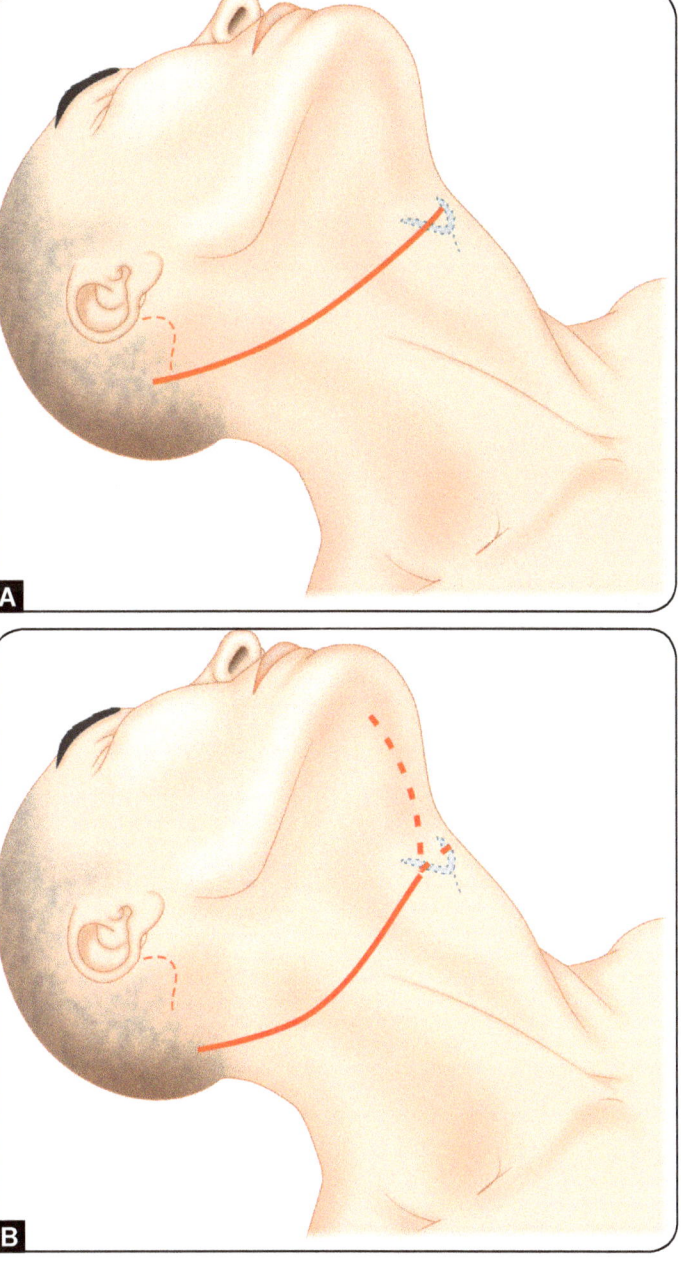

Figs. 5A and B

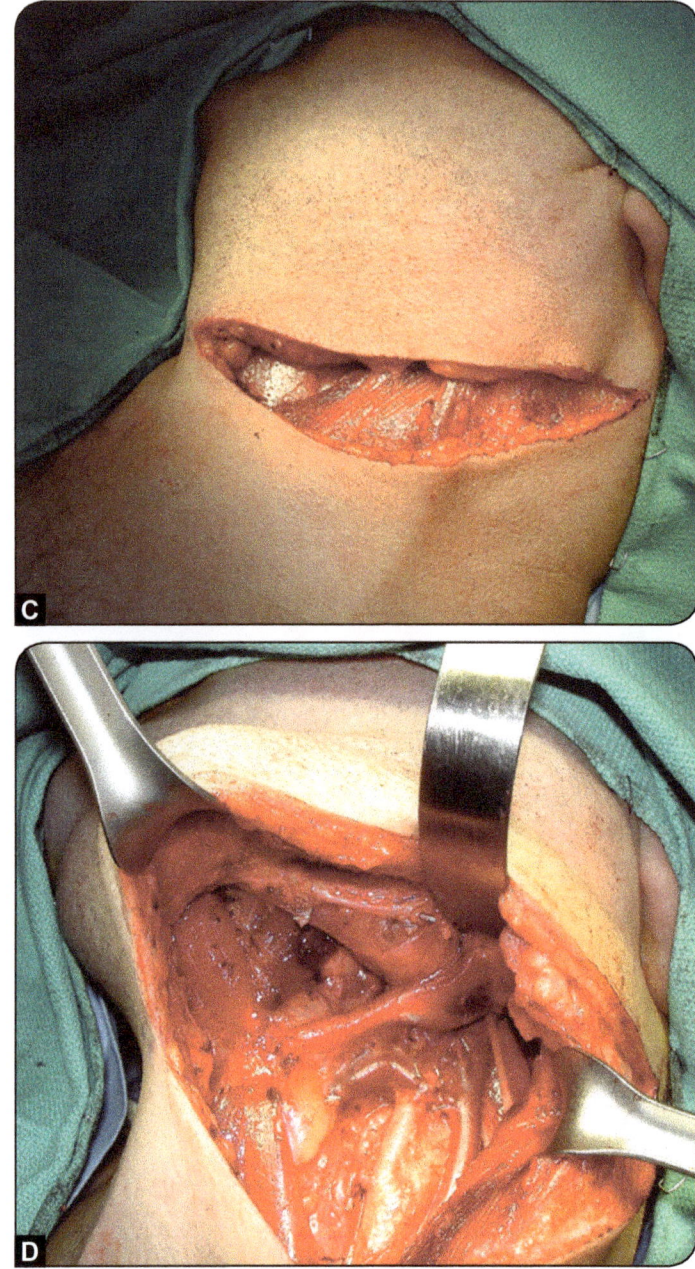

Figs. 5A to D: Upper transverse incision.

MIDNECK TRANSVERSE INCISION (FIGS. 6A AND B)

A. This incision is placed in a natural crease in the midlateral aspect of the neck. It provides enough exposure to perform an SND of levels II–IV. We have found this incision useful to perform an SND II–IV in the setting of a "planned" neck dissection after chemoradiotherapy.
B. Postoperative photograph showing the cosmetic results.

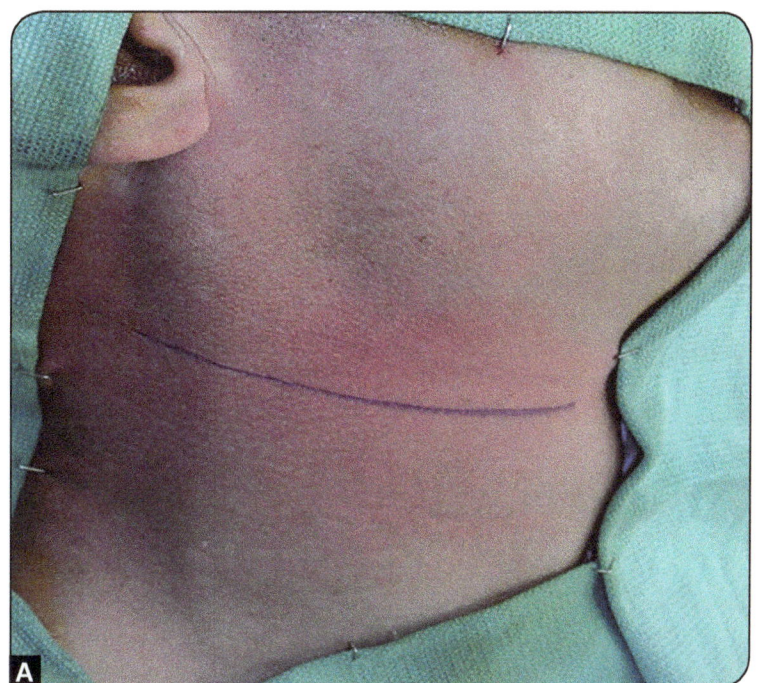

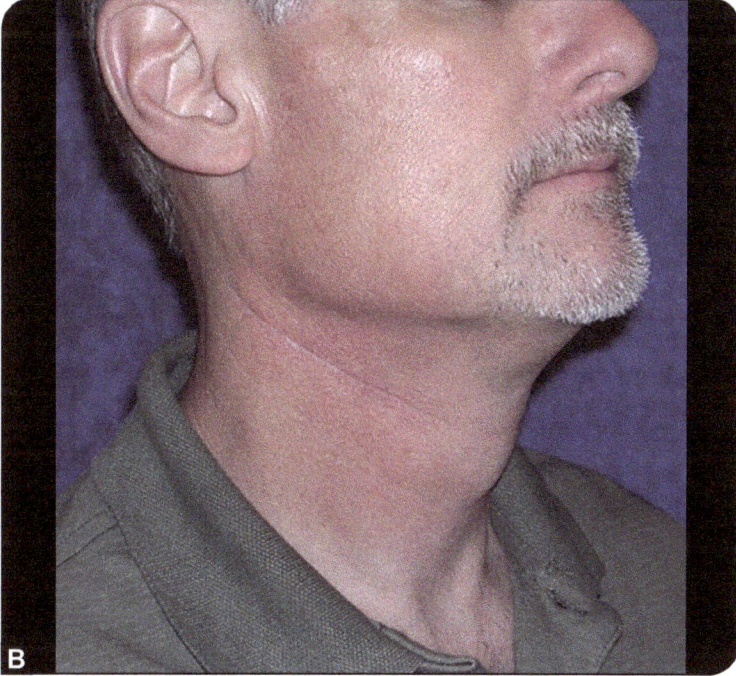

Figs. 6A and B: Midneck transverse incision.

LOW TRANSVERSE INCISION (FIGS. 7A TO C)

A. This incision is placed in a natural crease in the lower lateral aspect of the neck. It is often an extension of a thyroidectomy incision, posteriorly, up to the level of the anterior border of the trapezius. It is particularly useful when a neck dissection of levels II–V is performed in combination with a thyroidectomy.
B. Intraoperative photographs showing a modified radial neck dissection (MRND) with preservation of the SCMM, IJV and XIN and a thyroidectomy.
C. Postoperative photograph showing the cosmetic results.

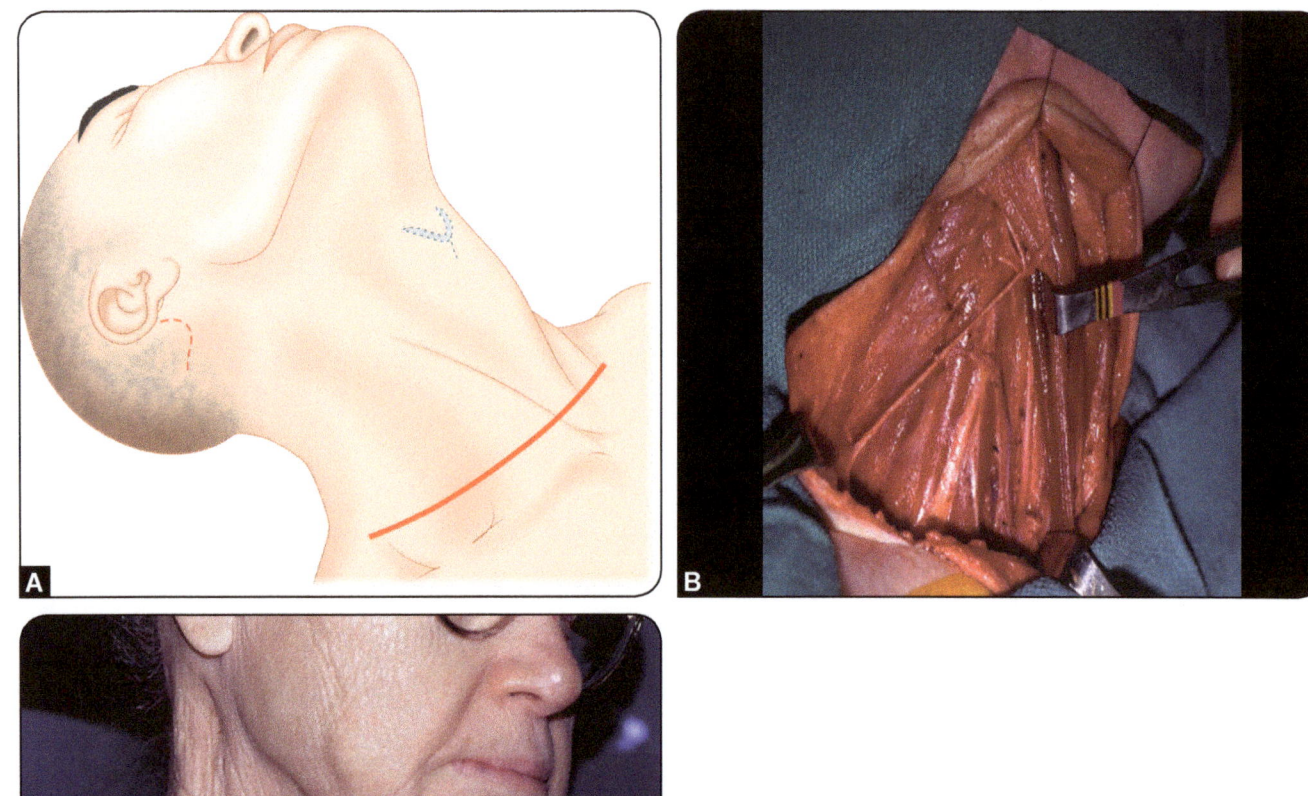

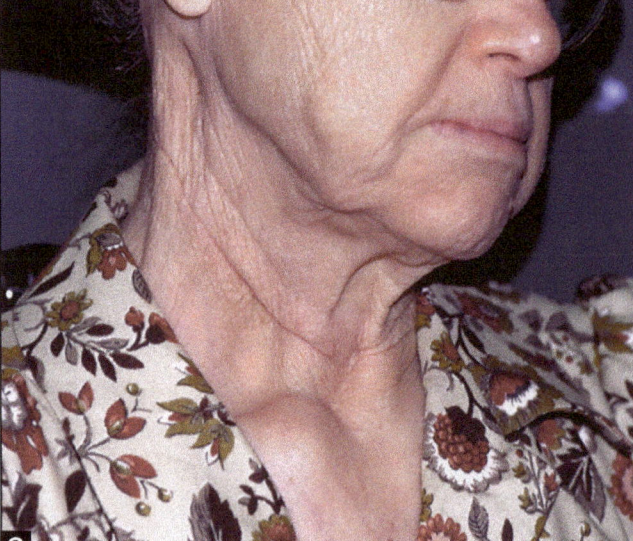

Figs. 7A to C: Low transverse incision.

UNILATERAL HOCKEY STICK INCISION (FIG. 8)

This incision extends obliquely down from about the level of the mastoid tip and curves forward about two finger breaths above the clavicle. It affords excellent exposure to perform a selective neck dissection of levels II–IV. Adding a descending limb, which extends obliquely down and backwards, provides access to the entire posterior triangle of the neck. Since the trifurcation is placed away from the carotid and the anterior inferior flap is very short, the postoperative viability of this flap is rarely, if ever, an issue.

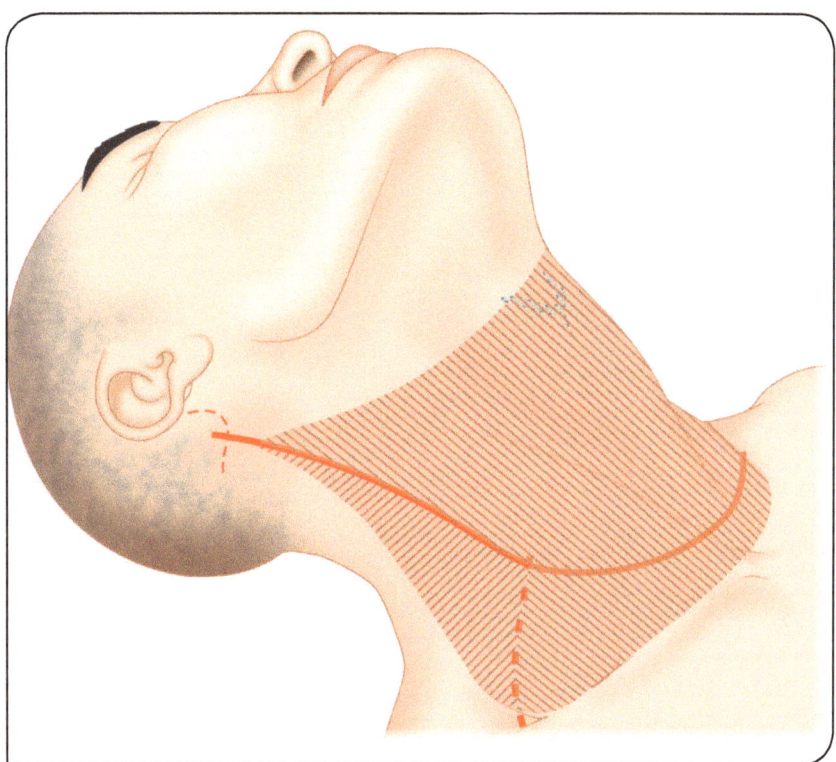

Fig. 8: Unilateral hockey stick incision. The areas of the neck easily accessible with this incision are shaded.

BILATERAL HOCKEY STICK INCISION OR LONG APRON-LIKE INCISION (FIG. 9)

This is the preferred incision to perform bilateral neck dissections with a total laryngectomy.

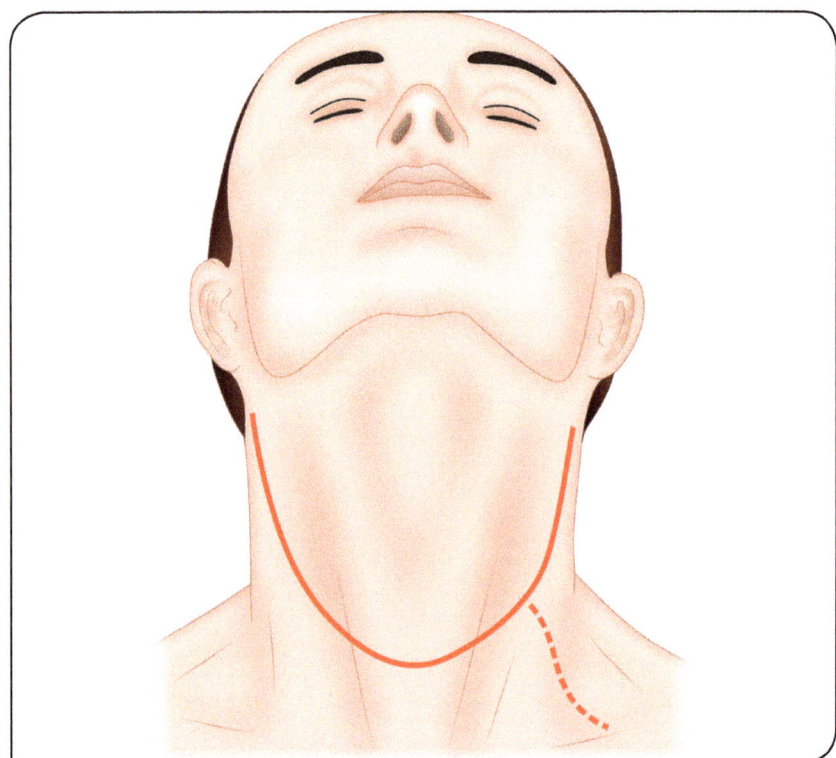

Fig. 9: Bilateral hockey stick incision or long apron-like incision.

CHAPTER 3

Radical Neck Dissection

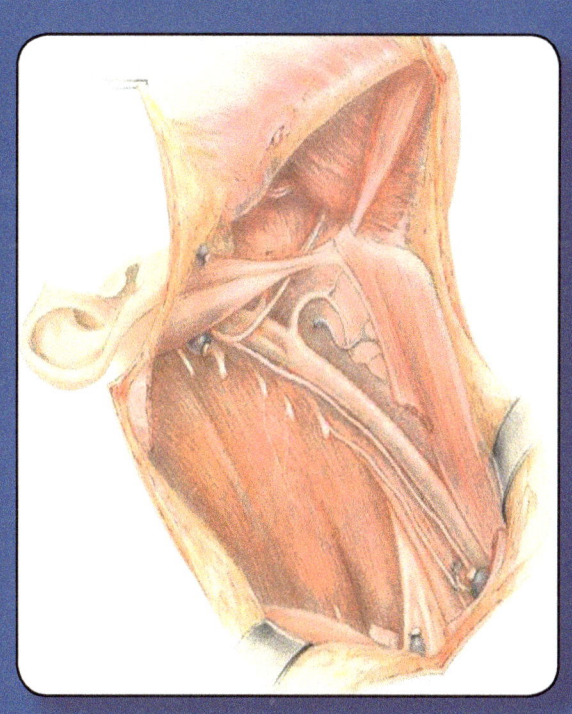

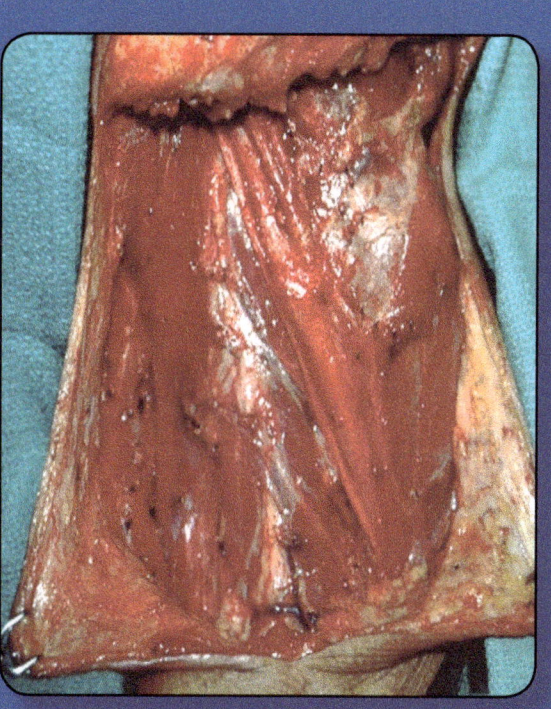

INTRODUCTION

The radical neck dissection (RND) removes lymph node groups I through V, the sternocleidomastoid muscle, the internal jugular vein and the spinal accessory nerve. The dissection extends from the inferior border of the mandible superiorly to the clavicle inferiorly, and from the anterior belly of the digastric muscle and the lateral border of the strap muscles, anteriorly, to the anterior border of the trapezius, posteriorly.

It appears that the first "RND" was performed in 1988 by a Polish surgeon by the name of Jawlensky. In that regard, Edward Towpik wrote in the Gazeta Lekarska in 1888,[1] "although not the first to perform the operation, Jawlensky was, to my knowledge, the first to describe the technique and extent of radical en bloc neck dissection. Published in a Polish medical journal, his contribution remained virtually unknown abroad. Jawlensky himself was apparently not aware of the true importance of his operation; he never mentioned its potential application in removing lymph node metastases".

The first description of a systematic block-like removal of the lymphatics of the neck for lymph node metastases was published by Crile in 1906.[2] The operation he described has come to be known as the RND which, as conceptualized above, removes the spinal accessory nerve. Interestingly, however, the drawings that illustrate Crile's publication depict the spinal accessory nerve and the ansa hypoglossi being preserved (Fig. 1).

Removal of the spinal accessory nerve during cervical lymphadenectomy was actually advocated several decades later as a means to decrease operating time and, more importantly, to assure a complete removal of the cervical lymph nodes.[3] The latter concept was championed and popularized in the 1950s by Martin,[4] who stated, "Any technique that is designed to preserve the spinal accessory nerve should be condemned unequivocally." As Chief of the Head and Neck Surgery Service at Memorial Sloan Kettering, Martin was very influential at the time. As a result, the RND was considered for many years the only acceptable operation for the treatment of the neck in patients with cancer.

Unfortunately, the resection of the spinal accessory nerve often results in disabling shoulder pain and decreased range of motion. In addition, when the operation is performed on both sides of the neck simultaneously, and

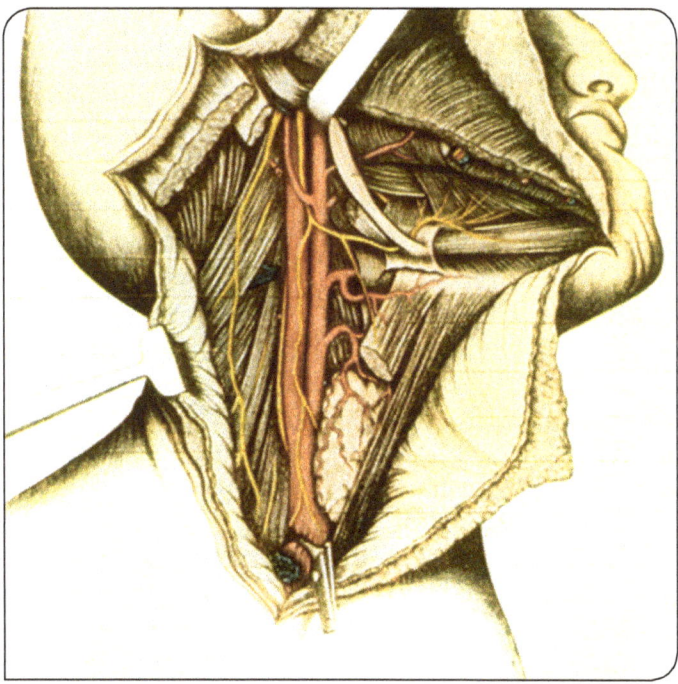

Fig. 1: Illustration of Crile's description of the RND. Note that the XI nerve, and the ansa hypoglossi, are shown preserved. *Source*: Reprinted with permission from Crile G. Excision of cancer of the head and neck. JAMA. 1906;47:1780-86.

sometimes even years apart, resection of both IJVs can lead to inappropriate secretion of antidiuretic hormone (ADH), brain edema and disfiguring facial lymphedema.[5] These observations prompted surgeons in the 1940s to begin preserving the spinal accessory nerve and, subsequently, to other modifications of the RND.

Indications

1. Multiple cervical lymph node metastases, particularly if some of the involved nodes are located in the posterior triangle of the neck around the spinal accessory nerve.
2. A large metastatic tumor mass or multiple matted nodes in the upper portion of the neck with obvious clinical, radiological or intraoperative evidence of involvement of the SCMM, the spinal accessory nerve or both.
3. When a neck dissection is performed to remove residual disease in the neck following an ill-advised incisional biopsy of a neck node containing metastatic tumor. In some such cases, extensive undermining during the biopsy procedure, postoperative inflammation and ecchymosis, often obscure the relation of the tumor to the SCMM, spinal accessory nerve, or IJV making their preservation problematic.

SURGICAL TECHNIQUE

The patient is positioned on the operating table with the neck extended, if necessary, with a roll under the shoulders, the head turned towards the opposite side and stabilized with a foam doughnut.

The incisions most commonly used to perform a RND are discussed in Chapter 2. The choice of the incision depends mainly on the location of the primary tumor, the length of the neck and on whether a portion of skin of the neck needs to be resected. For instance, an apron-like incision may be the choice when a RND is to be done in conjunction with a total laryngectomy. If a metastatic node in the submandibular area is extensive enough that the overlying skin has to be resected, an elliptical incision around the tumor in the neck can be combined with a modified Schobinger incision.

Skin flaps are elevated in a subplatysmal plane. However, depending upon the size and extent of the tumor in the neck, the platysma may be left over the area involved by tumor as the skin flaps are elevated in a supraplatysmal plane.

Dissection of the Submandibular and Submental Triangles

Steps of dissection of the submandibular and submental triangles are as follows:

- *2A*: As the superior neck flap is elevated, it is important to keep the plane of dissection superficial to the fascia that covers the submandibular gland (superficial layer of the deep cervical fascia). If the gland is exposed at this point, the plane of dissection is too deep and identification of the ramus mandibularis may be difficult. "Pushing" (not pinching) the upper flap or platysma upwards facilitates elevation of the flap in the right plain.
- *2B*: Identification of the ramus mandibularis is a necessary step to preserve this nerve while removing the prevascular and retrovascular submandibular lymph nodes. A useful maneuver is to have the assistant surgeon flatten the tissues of the area by pressing gently on them with three or four fingers spread above the level of the inferior border of the mandible. The surgeon places three or four fingers about 1 cm below the assistant's. The surgeon and the assistant then move their fingers up and down in a coordinated fashion, sliding the submandibular fascia over the gland and over the inferior border of the mandible. Sliding the fascia in this manner usually enables the surgeon to see the "shadow" of the submandibular gland through it and, in some cases, to see the ramus mandibularis through the fascia above the gland; the fascia is incised 1–2 mm above the perceived superior border of the gland, starting about 4–5 mm in front and below the angle of the mandible. This incision is very "shallow" and extends forward 1.5–2 cm in a direction parallel to the inferior border of the mandible.

  The assistant surgeon moves his or her fingers closer to the upper edge of the incised fascia and gently pushes it upward, while the surgeon does the same to the inferior cut edge, but in the opposite direction. Small vessels are controlled with bipolar cautery to maintain a bloodless field. These maneuvers are repeated two or more times until the nerve is clearly visualized.

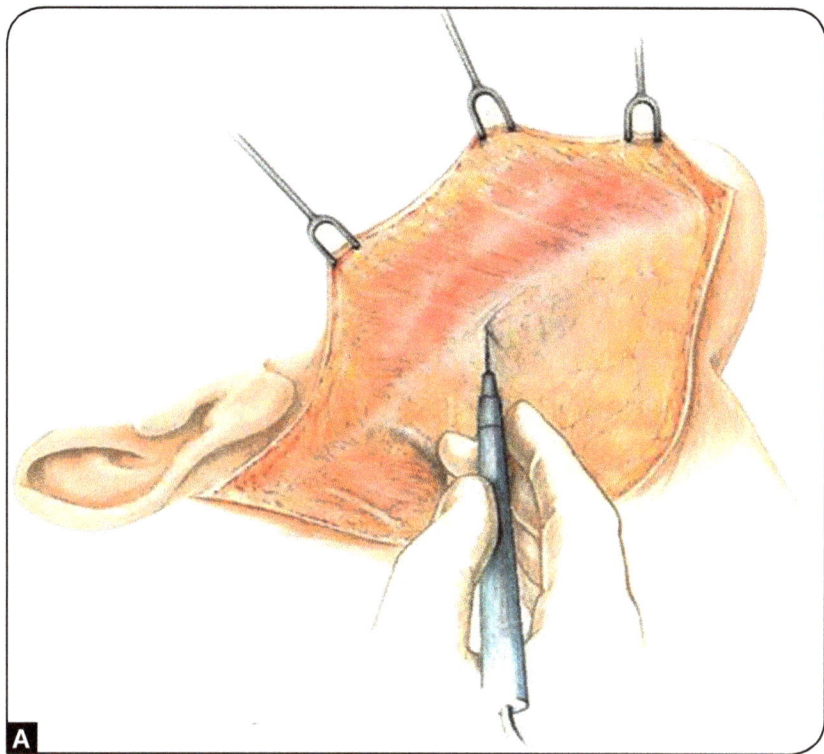

Fig. 2A

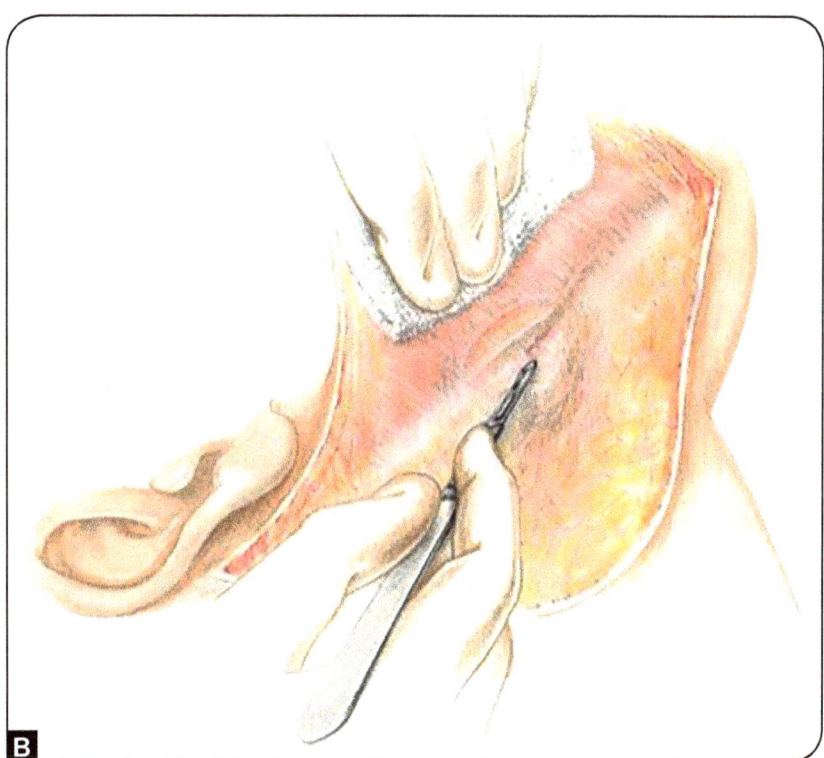

Fig. 2B

- *2C*: The ramus mandibularis lies deep to the fascia but superficial to the facial vessels, which are exposed below the level of the nerve with blunt dissection; the fatty tissue that surrounds them is divided. The submandibular prevascular and retrovascular lymph nodes, which are usually immediately below or medial to the nerve, are likewise exposed. When these nodes are involved by tumor, it is preferable to leave the platysma attached to them. In such cases, it may not be possible, nor desirable, to expose and preserve the ramus mandibularis.

- *2D*: When these submandibular nodes are not involved by tumor, or if they are small and clearly separable from the nerve, the nerve is preserved and the nodes are carefully dissected away from it. In doing so, the facial vessels are exposed and divided. Notice the prevascular node in front of the facial artery and the retrovascular node behind the facial vein.

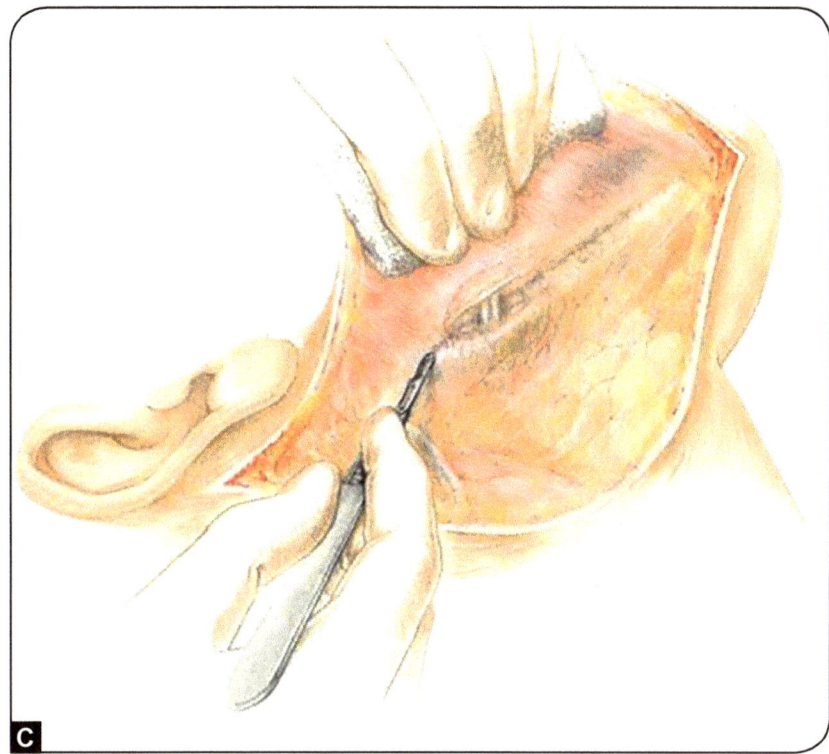

Fig. 2C

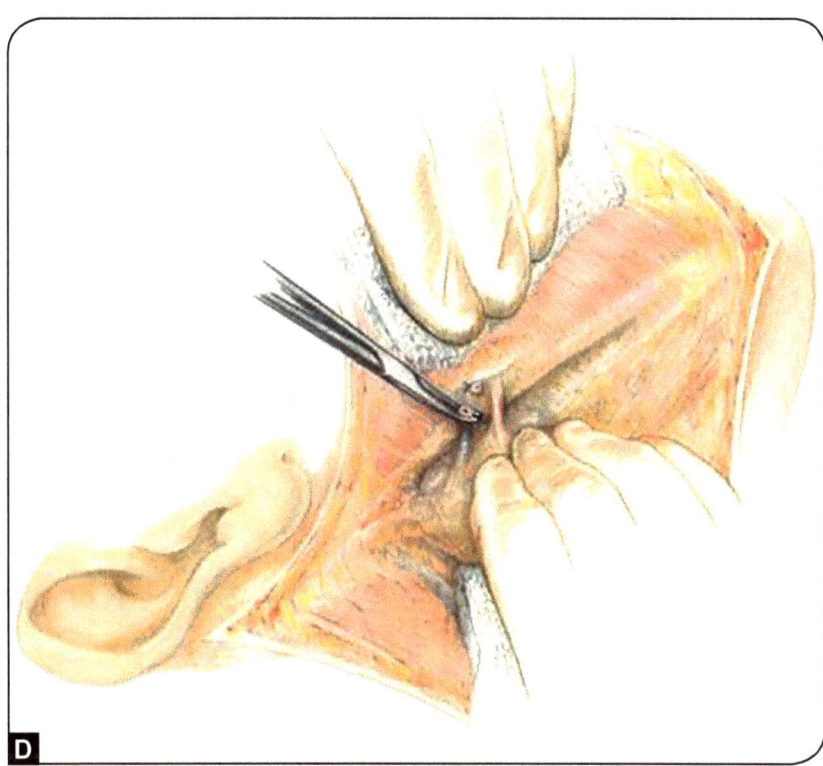

Fig. 2D

- *2E:* The next step is to incise the fascia and fatty tissues along the inferior border of the mandible and continue the dissection through the lax connective tissue medial to the mandible. As this proceeds, it is usually necessary or preferable to identify and divide two structures: (1) the submental artery (a branch of the facial artery) located deep within the fatty tissue in the angle between the anterior belly of the digastric and the inferior border of the mandible, and (2) the nerve to the mylohyoid, usually found between the posterior border of the mylohyoid and the angle of the mandible. A small artery, a vein or both usually accompany the nerve. It is advisable to ligate, clip or cauterize these vessels before dividing them because they can retract upwards, under the mandible and cause bleeding that is cumbersome to control. Once this is done, and if the location and extent of the primary tumor does not preclude it, the surgeon should be able to place a fingertip behind and above the posterior-superior aspect of the submandibular gland and gently push it forward and downward. This should be easy to do because the tissue around the gland here is very lax. Doing this establishes a plane lateral to the hyoglossus muscle, which facilitates later exposure and division of the submandibular ganglion and duct, while leaving the hypoglossal nerve and accompanying veins undisturbed.

- *2F:* At this point, if the operation is to include the submental triangle, the superior flap must be elevated up to the inferior border of the mandible in the midline. The dissection of the submental triangle begins at the superior "apex" of the triangle, immediately below the mandible, between the superior insertion of the anterior belly of the digastric muscles. Usually, there is a small artery that courses upward at this point and it may need to be ligated or clipped. Then, the tissue at the apex is grasped with a forceps and it is dissected downward. A lymph node is usually located very near the apex of triangle, thus, the importance of including this area in the dissection. The fatty tissue of the submental triangle is dissected off of the anterior belly of the digastric muscles and the mylohyoid, down to the level of the hyoid bone. The fibro-fatty tissue in this area can be several millimeters thick and can house lymph nodes that may be involved by tumor in patients with cancer of the lower lip and the anterior floor of the mouth.

  If, on the other hand, the submental triangle is not included in the dissection, the dissection of the submandibular triangle begins by incising the fascia and fibro-fatty tissues along the anterior belly of the digastric muscle.

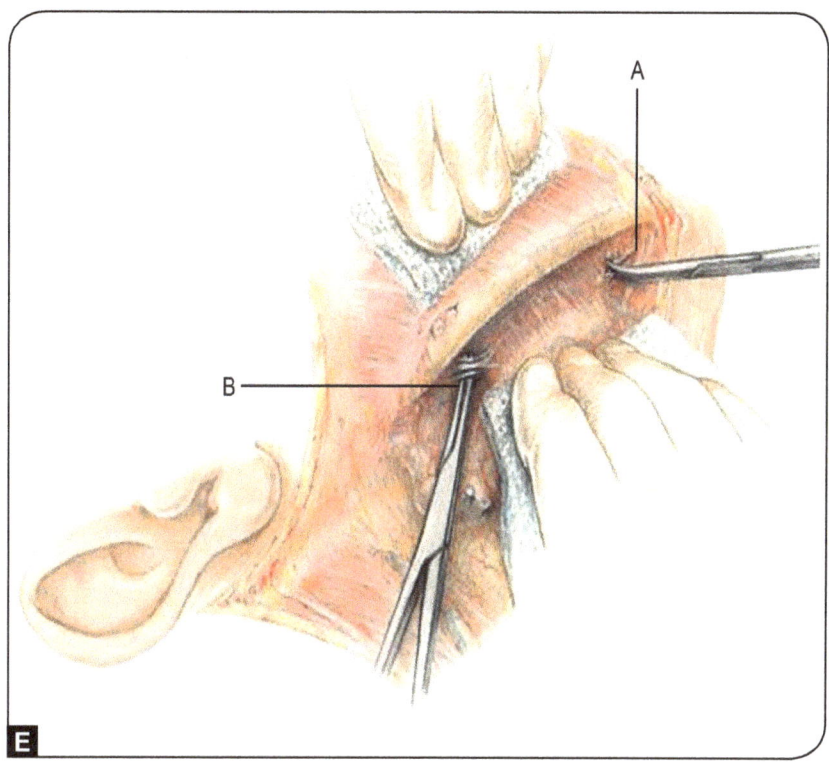

Fig. 2E: (A) Submental artery. (B) Nerve to the mylohyoid.

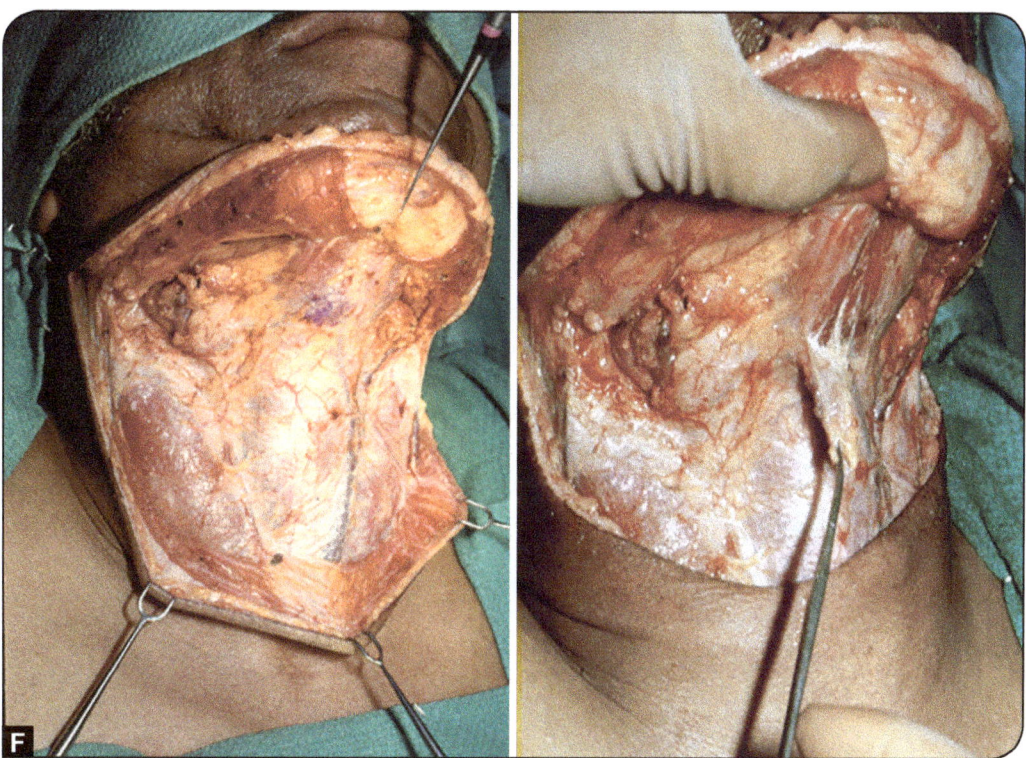

Fig. 2F

- *2G:* The fascia is then dissected off of the anterior belly of the ipsilateral digastric muscle, as the specimen is retracted posteriorly, removing the fibrous fatty tissue containing lymph nodes lateral to the mylohyoid muscle. A "clean" dissection of this area is important because it contains the preglandular lymph node(s), which can be the first echelon of lymphatic drainage for the floor of the mouth and oral tongue.

- *2H:* When the dissection reaches the posterior border of the mylohyoid, this muscle is retracted forward (with a Richardson or a Greene retractor). This exposes three structures that are somewhat parallel but in different planes; from lateral to medial and from top to bottom they are: (1) the lingual nerve, (2) the submandibular gland duct and (3) the hypoglossal nerve.
  The lingual nerve and the submandibular ganglion extending downward from it are clearly seen. The ganglion can then be easily divided.

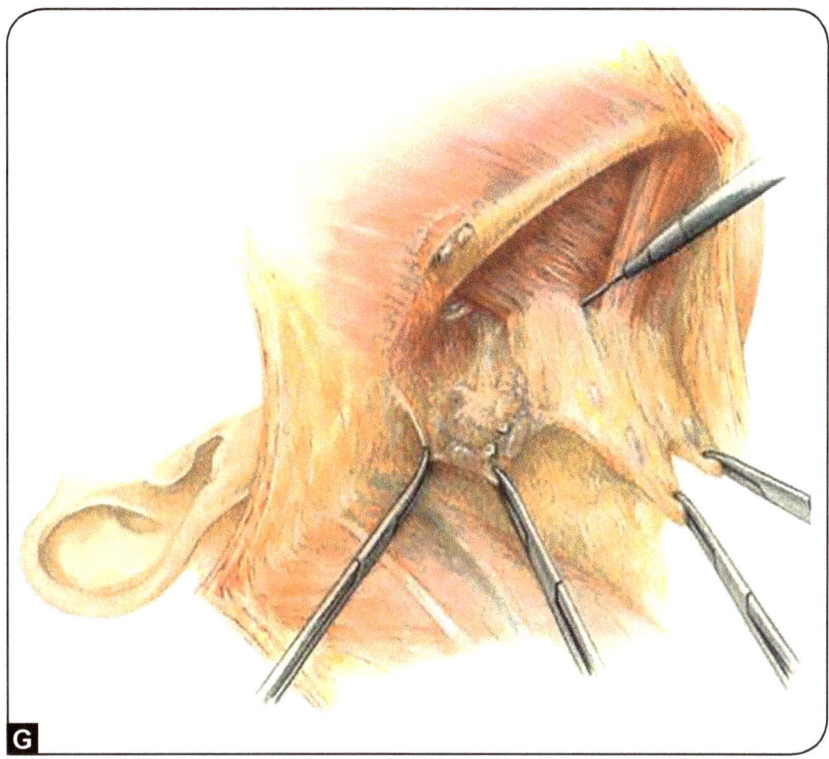

Fig. 2G

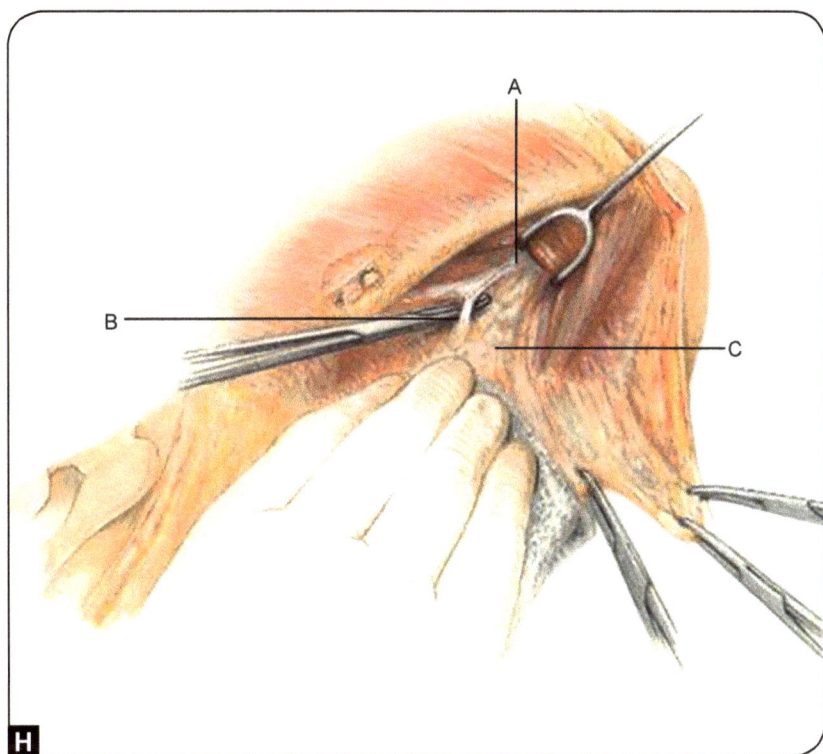

Fig. 2H: (A) Lingual nerve. (B) Submandibular ganglion. (C) Submandibular duct.

- *2I:* Next, the duct of the submandibular gland is exposed and divided. Pushing with one finger the lax tissues medial to these structures, along the previously established plane lateral to the hyoglossus muscle, decreases the likelihood of inadvertent injury to the hypoglossal nerve while dividing them; the hypoglossal nerve and the veins that accompany it are not easily displaced laterally. Notice the hypoglossal nerve deep or medial to the duct, which is being lifted with a hemostat prior to being divided.

- *2J:* The contents of the submandibular triangle are now freed up anteriorly and can then be easily dissected off of the hyoglossus muscle and the digastric tendon in a posterior direction. In doing so, the hypoglossal and its accompanying veins are not disturbed. As the specimen is retracted posteriorly, the facial artery is pulled over the posterior belly of the digastric muscle, which facilitates its division between clamps. The dissection of the submandibular triangle is thus completed.

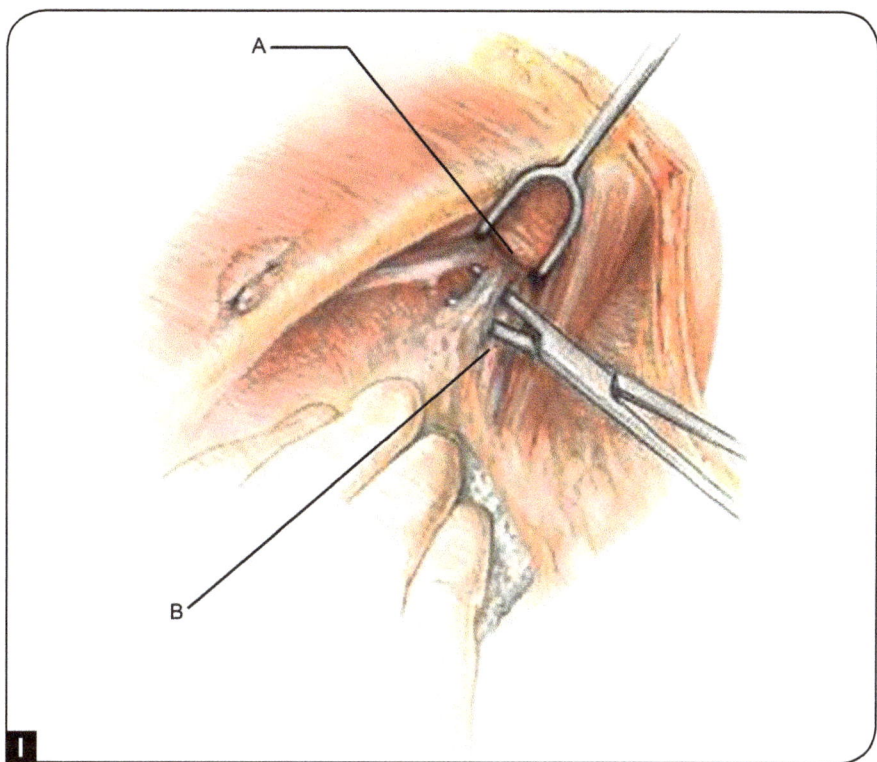

Fig. 2I: (A) Submandibular duct. (B) Hypoglossal nerve.

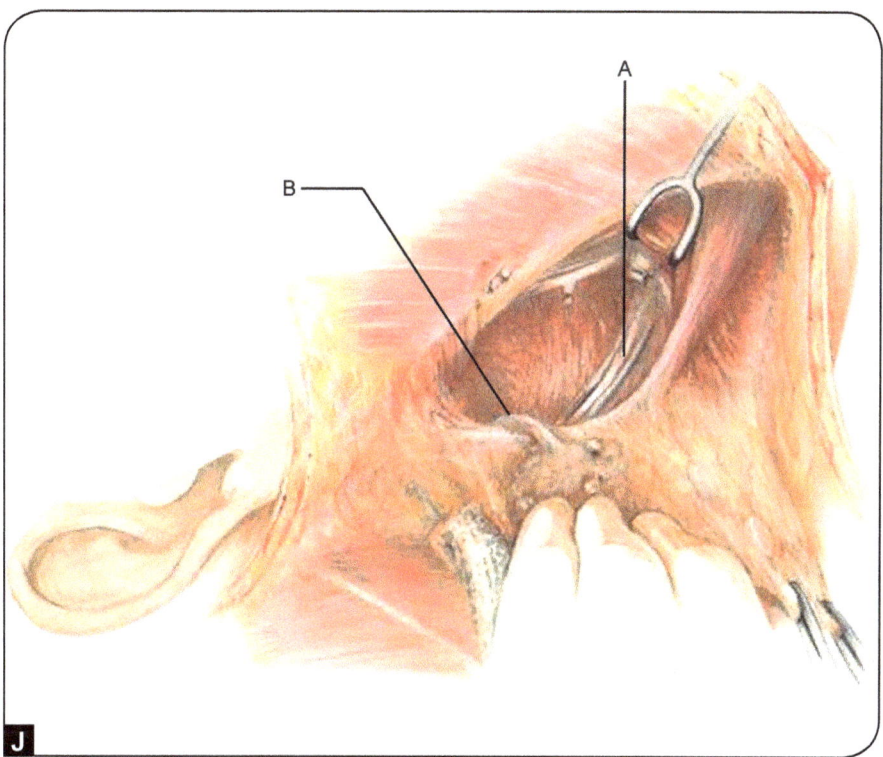

Fig. 2J: (A) Hypoglossal nerve and vena comitans. (B) Facial artery.

Superior Lateral Dissection

This portion of the neck dissection is crucial since the majority of metastases occur to the nodes in this level; also, the majority of recurrences after neck dissection occur in this area of the neck. Therefore, it is important to do this part pristinely, avoiding transecting any lymph node and, more importantly, avoiding getting too close to or entering the lymph node obviously involved by metastatic tumor.

Depending upon the location and the size of the nodes involved by tumor in the upper portion of the neck, the tail of the parotid gland may be dissected and retracted superiorly or transected if necessary to provide an adequate tissue margin. Likewise, it may be necessary to include the posterior belly of the digastric in the dissected specimen. If the digastric does not need to be removed, it is slightly retracted upwards with an Army-Navy or a similar retractor.

- *3A:* In either case, it is prudent to identify next the upper most portion of the IJV, the spinal accessory nerve and the hypoglossal nerve. A useful technique to accomplish this safely consists of applying gentle inferior traction to the "specimen" and using a fine tip hemostat, such as a mosquito clamp, to facilitate incising the fascia and soft tissues of the region. To do this, it is essential for the tissues of the area to be reasonably flattened by the surgeon's fingers; then, the surgeon applies the tip of the mosquito clamp to the tissues and, using fine dissecting motion and the necessary pressure, pierces a thin layer of tissue. Changing the angle of the clamp as needed, the surgeon drives the tip of the clamp in a posterior direction. Opening the clamp a few millimeters and elevating with it a see-through layer of tissue allows cutting it without risk of injuring the underlying structures. This maneuver is repeated, along the length of the digastric, as needed to expose the desired structures. More often than not, this part of the dissection requires ligating or clipping small branches of the occipital artery that course toward the SCMM and small tributaries of the IJV. When these vessels are torn, hurried efforts to control the bleeding by clamping attempts in a bloody field jeopardize the hypoglossal nerve.

- *3B:* The hypoglossal nerve as well as the superior most portions of the IJV and the spinal accessory nerve are exposed.

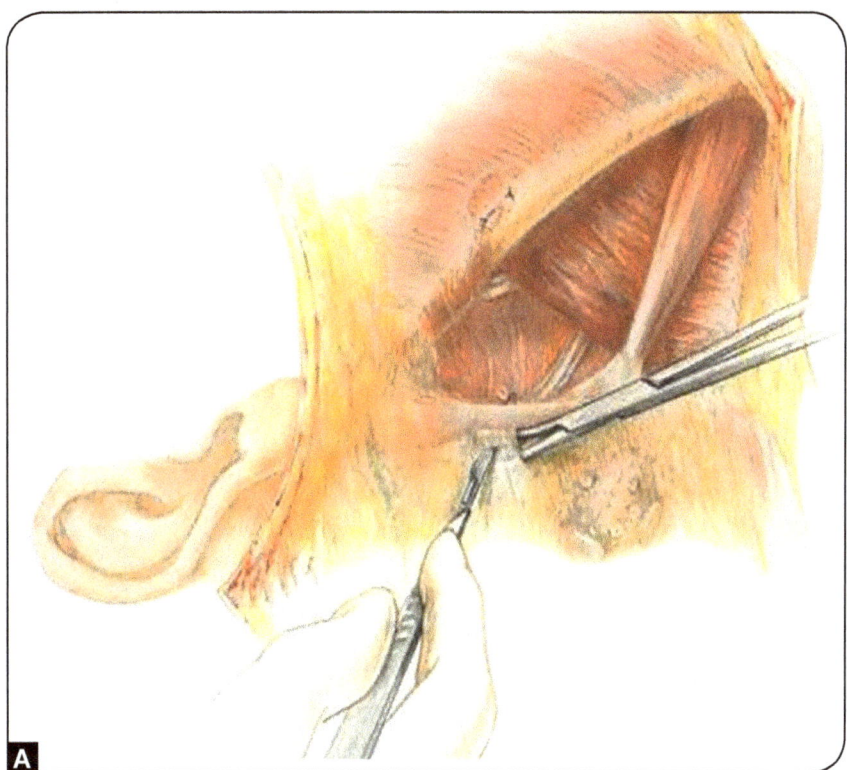

Fig. 3A

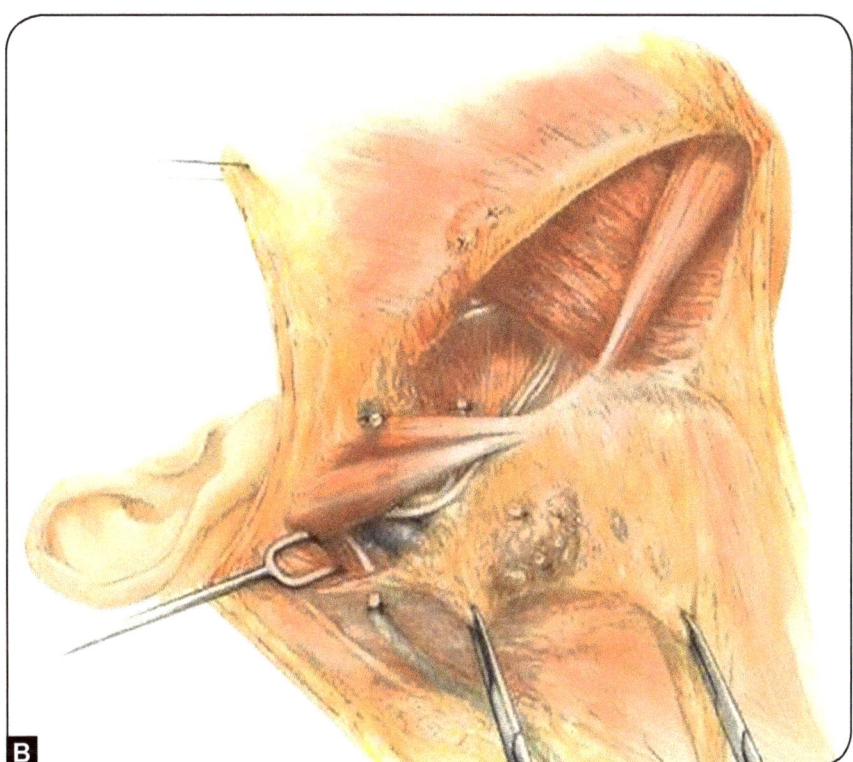

Fig. 3B

- *3C:* The next step consists of dividing the external jugular vein and the greater auricular nerve as they enter the parotid gland. Then, the SCMM is incised close to its insertion in the mastoid process. It should be kept in mind that, at this level, the muscle is thick and tendinous anteriorly and thinner posteriorly. This step can be performed either before or after the steps described in 3A.

- *3D:* The fibro-fatty tissue medial to the SCMM is incised, preferably beginning posteriorly where this layer is usually very thin and then proceeding anteriorly. In this manner, the splenius capitis muscle posteriorly and the levator scapulae muscle anteriorly are exposed.

  The spinal accessory nerve is transected. When the nerve is adjacent to or it is encased by an involved node attention should be paid to the appearance and diameter of the nerve. A thickened nerve that has a rather pinkish colour is suspicious for the presence of perineural tumor invasion. In that case, the transected end of the nerve should be submitted for frozen section examination. Otherwise, if it is at all possible, the uppermost portion of the nerve is dissected so that a small portion of the nerve can be preserved to allow nerve grafting after the specimen is removed.

  If a metastatic tumor mass is located low in the jugulodigastric region or in the midjugular region, the IJV is first ligated and divided superiorly. Otherwise, it may be preferable to leave this area alone and ligate the IJV low in the neck first. For instance, if the tumor is located high in the jugulodigastric region, especially if it is extensive and may require removal of the external carotid artery or the hypoglossal nerve, the IJV is divided inferiorly and the dissection is carried in a superior direction along the common carotid artery. By doing so, mobilization of the surgical specimen allows easier dissection of it from the internal carotid artery and, if possible, the external carotid artery and the hypoglossal nerve.

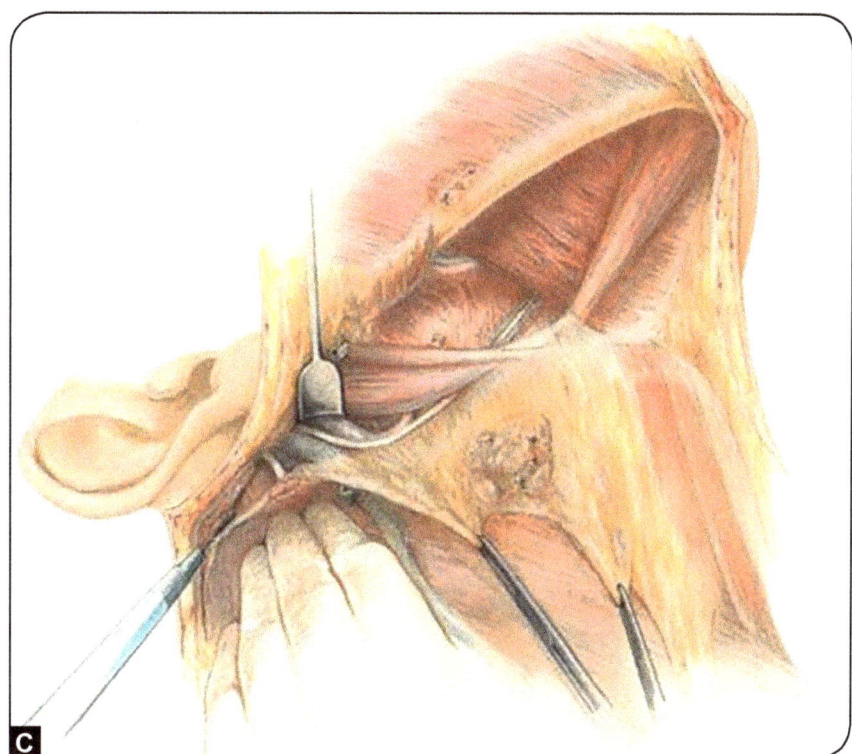

Fig. 3C

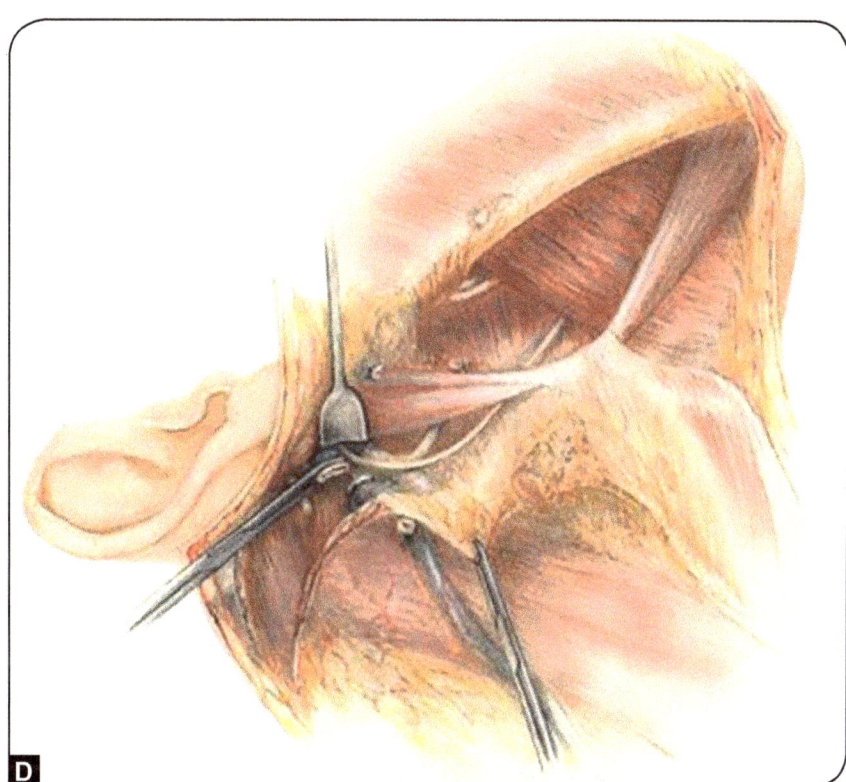

Fig. 3D

Posterior Dissection

Steps of posterior dissection are as follows:

- *4A:* The dissection is continued posteriorly and inferiorly along the anterior border of the trapezius muscle. The fibro-fatty tissue of the posterior triangle of the neck is then dissected forward and downward in a plane immediately lateral to the fascia of the splenius and the levator scapulae muscles. The spinal accessory nerve and the transverse cervical vessels are divided inferiorly as they cross the anterior border of the trapezius muscle.

- *4B:* During this portion of the operation, it is important to preserve the nerves to the levator scapulae muscle, unless the extent of the disease in the neck precludes it. These are two or more branches of the cervical plexus that run obliquely, laterally and downward, in a plane immediately under the thin fascia that covers the muscle (arrows). Therefore, to preserve them, the dissection over the levator must be carried out in a plane immediately superficial to its fascia.

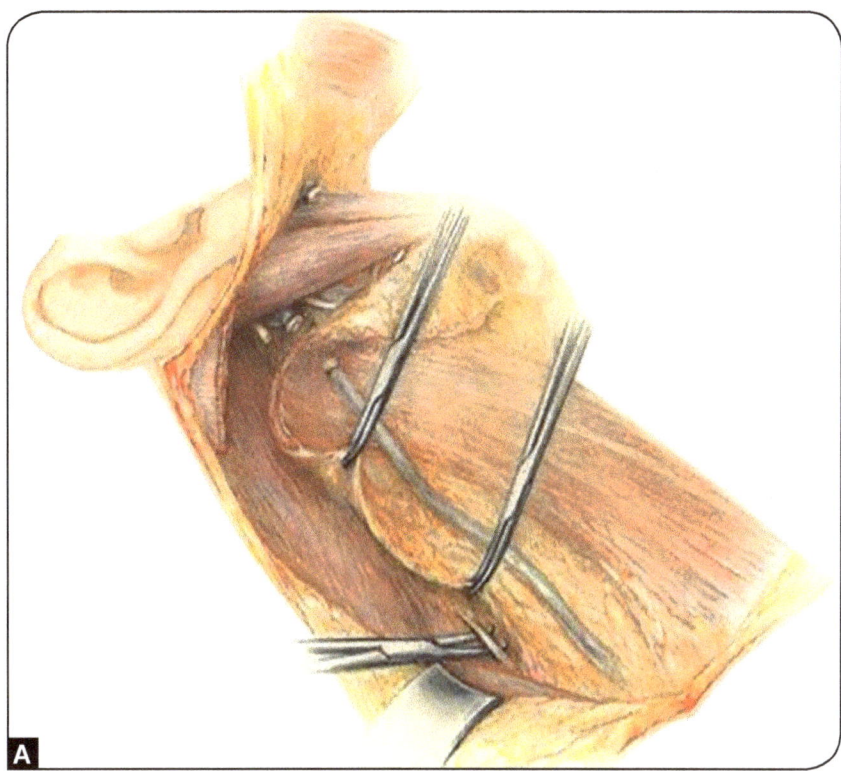

Fig. 4A: The spinal accessory nerve is exposed in front of the trapezius muscle prior to being divided.

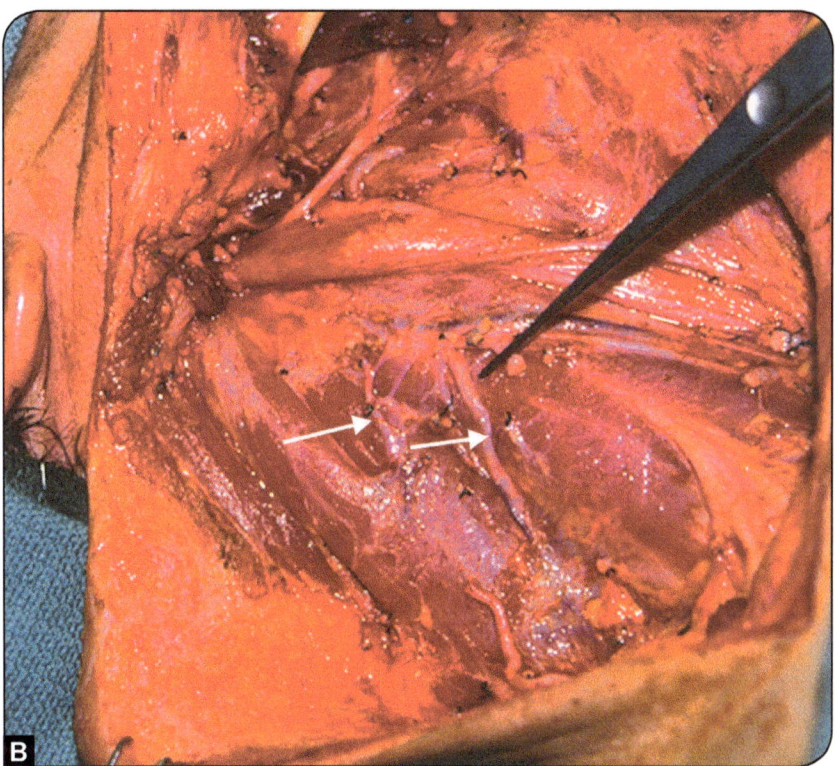

Fig. 4B: Arrows point to the nerves to the levator scapula.

Inferior Dissection

Steps of inferior dissection are as follows:

- *5A:* The SCMM is divided immediately above its inferior insertion in the clavicle and the sternum. Then, the superficial layer of the deep cervical fascia, medial and posterior to the muscle is incised above the superior border of the clavicle, in a layer-by-layer fashion.

- *5B:* Lateral to the insertion of the SCMM, the lower end of the external jugular vein and the omohyoid muscle are divided. Medially, the inferior end of the IJV may be ligated at this stage.

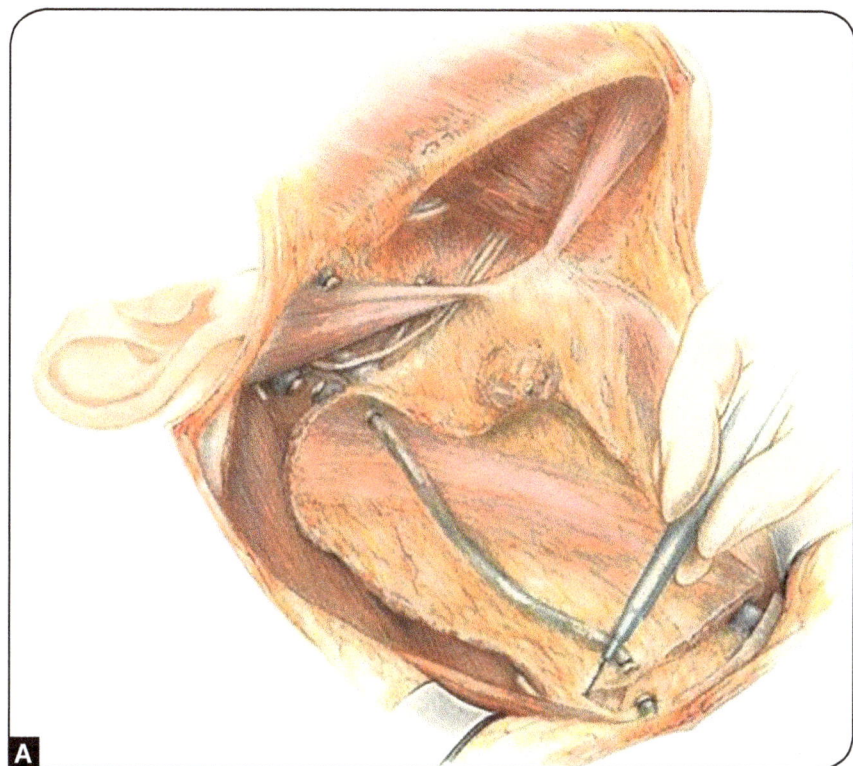

Fig. 5A

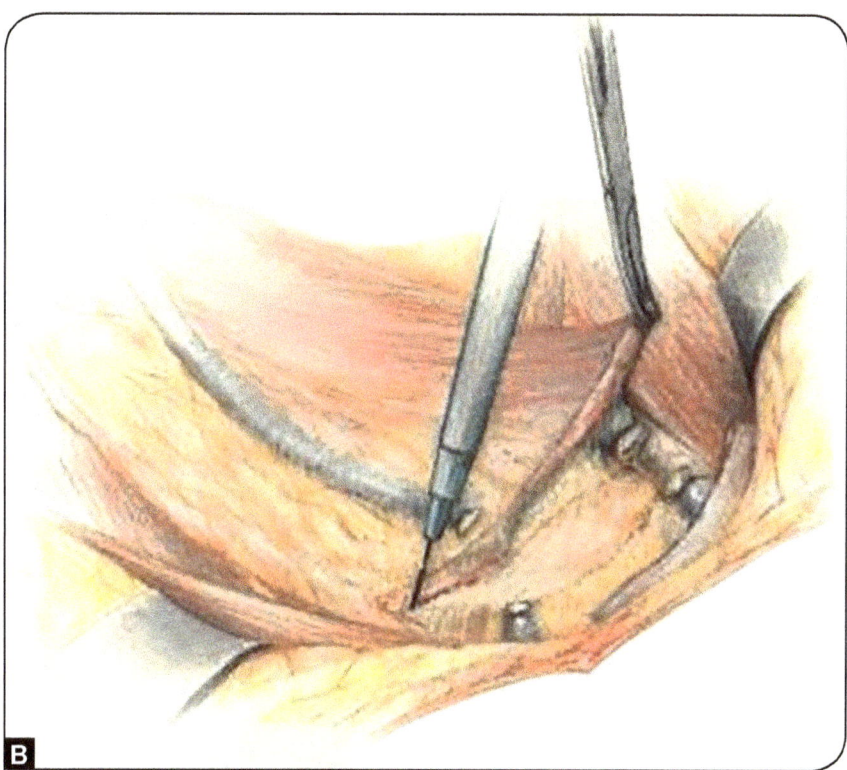

Fig. 5B

■ *5C:* After several *fascial* layers are incised, the fibro-fatty tissue in this region can be swept in an upward direction, exposing the brachial plexus, the scalenus muscles and the phrenic nerve.

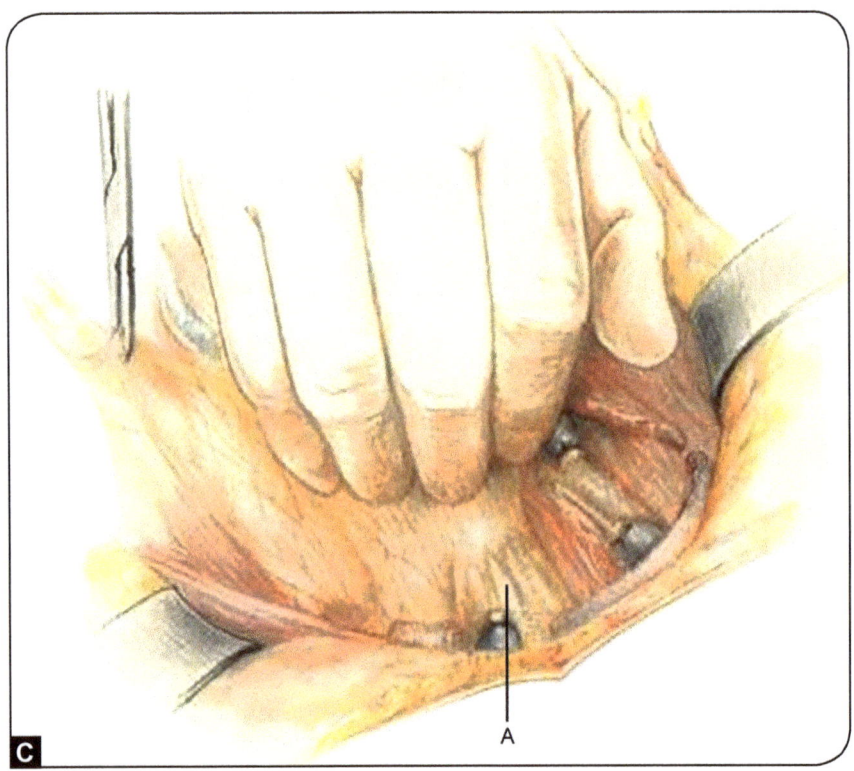

Fig. 5C: (A) Brachial plexus.

Medial Dissection

Steps of medial dissection are as follows:

■ *6A:* The dissection is now carried forward as the specimen is dissected off of the scalenus medius, the brachial plexus and the scalenus anticus. Care must be taken not to injure the phrenic nerve inferiorly (Fig. 6A). In the anterior inferior portion of the neck, the thoracic duct on the left side or an accessory duct on the right often needs to be ligated. The duct is anterior or superficial to the anterior scalene muscle and the phrenic nerve and posterior to the carotid and the vagus nerve. A diagram showing the anatomic relationship of the different structures of this area is shown in Figure 6B. To avoid a chyle leak through contributing lymphatic channels, the fat in this region is clipped using ligaclips and then cut.

As the dissection continues superiorly, the cutaneous branches of the cervical plexus are divided, preserving the nerves to the levator muscle. After this is done, only a relatively thin layer of tissue remains to be incised before the vagus nerve, the common carotid artery, and the IJV are exposed.

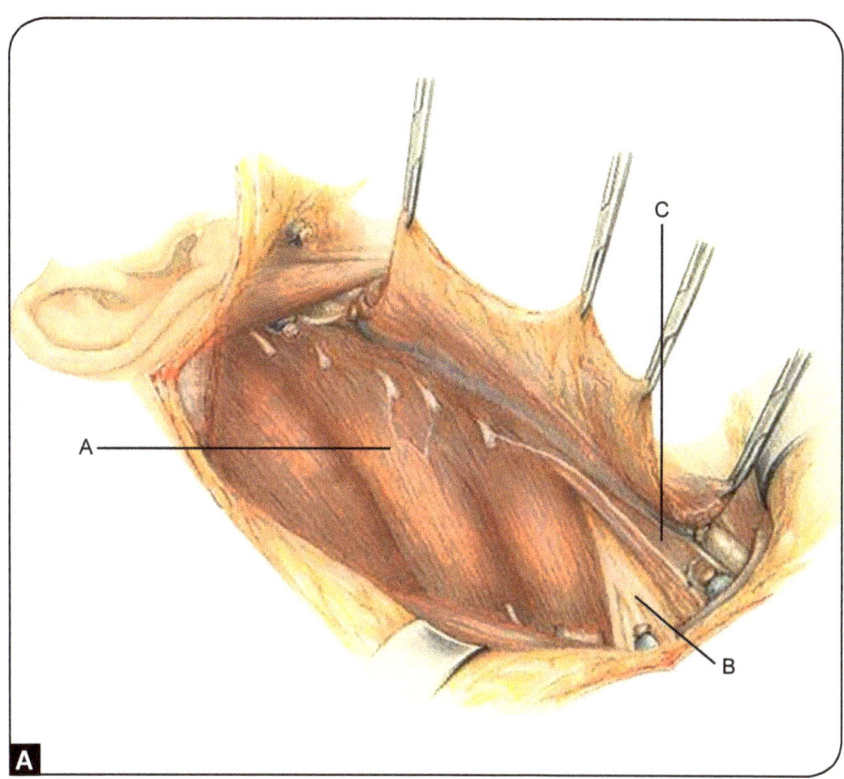

Fig. 6A: (A) Nerves to the levator scapulae muscle. (B) Brachial plexus. (C) Phrenic nerve.

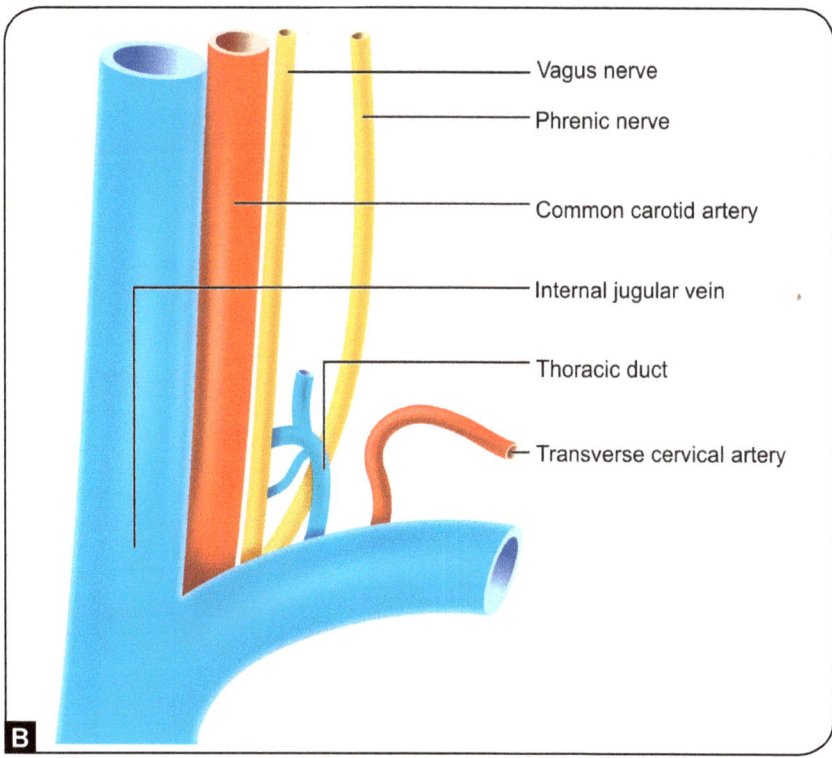

Vagus nerve

Phrenic nerve

Common carotid artery

Internal jugular vein

Thoracic duct

Transverse cervical artery

Fig. 6B

- *6C:* The dissection is then carried in a plane between the posterior medial aspect of the IJV and the vagus nerve and the common carotid artery. The medial end of the dissection is the lateral border of the strap muscles. As seen in the figure, at this stage, the anterior "belly" of the omohyoid muscle is divided.

- *6D:* As the dissection continues superiorly and usually below the level of the hypoglossal nerve, the superior thyroid, common facial and lingual veins are encountered and must be divided and ligated. More often than not, these veins drain into the IJV in a variety of combined ways; in Figure 6D, a common thyro-facial-lingual vein is being divided. Needless to say that during this portion of the operation, care must be taken to protect and preserve the hypoglossal nerve.

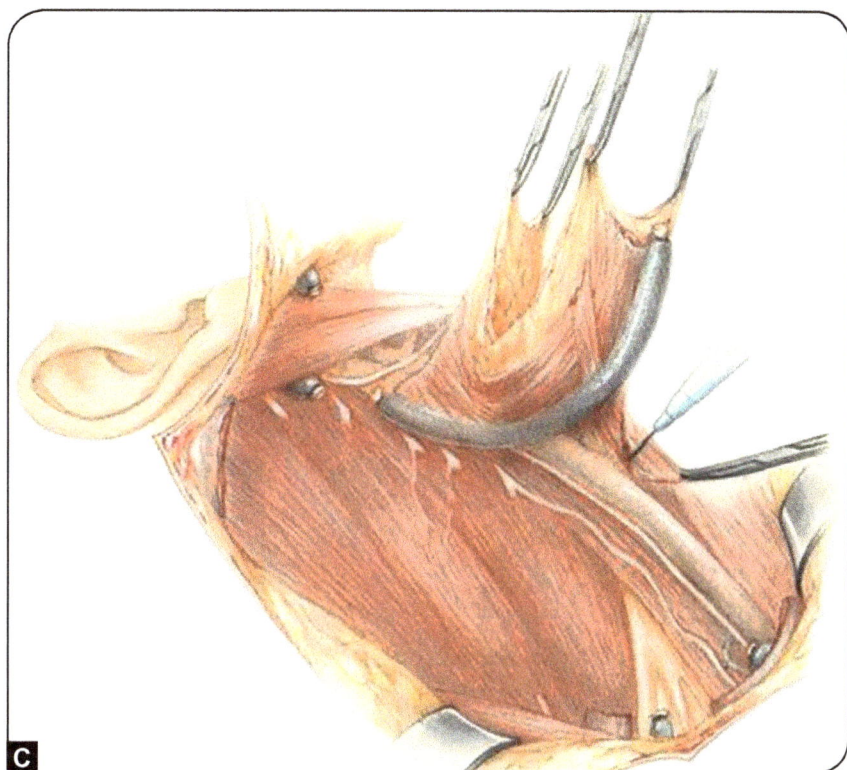

Fig. 6C

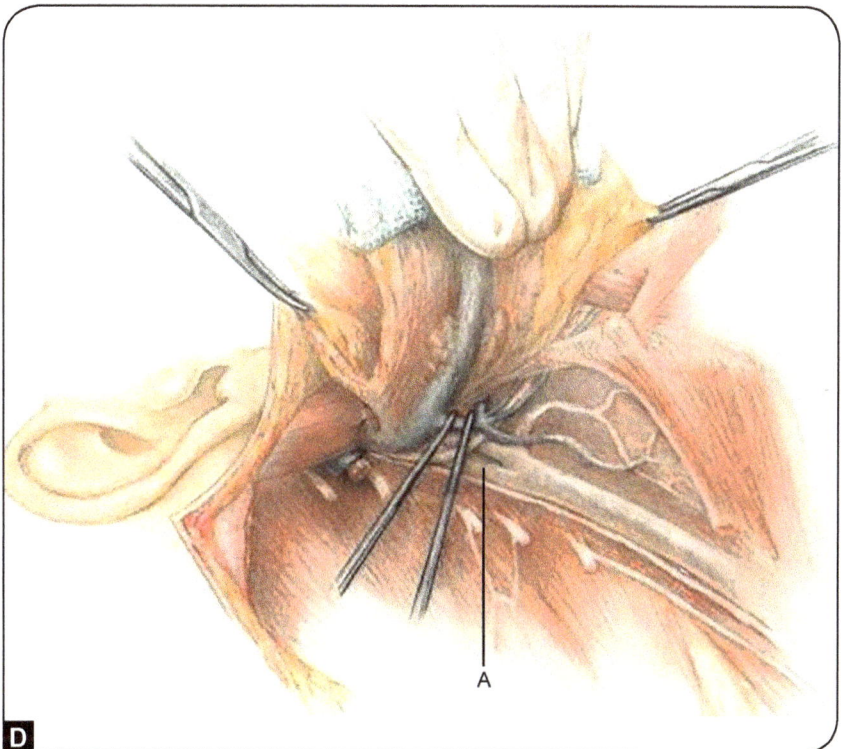

Fig. 6D: (A) Hypoglossal nerve.

- *6E:* The completed dissection section is shown in this figure.

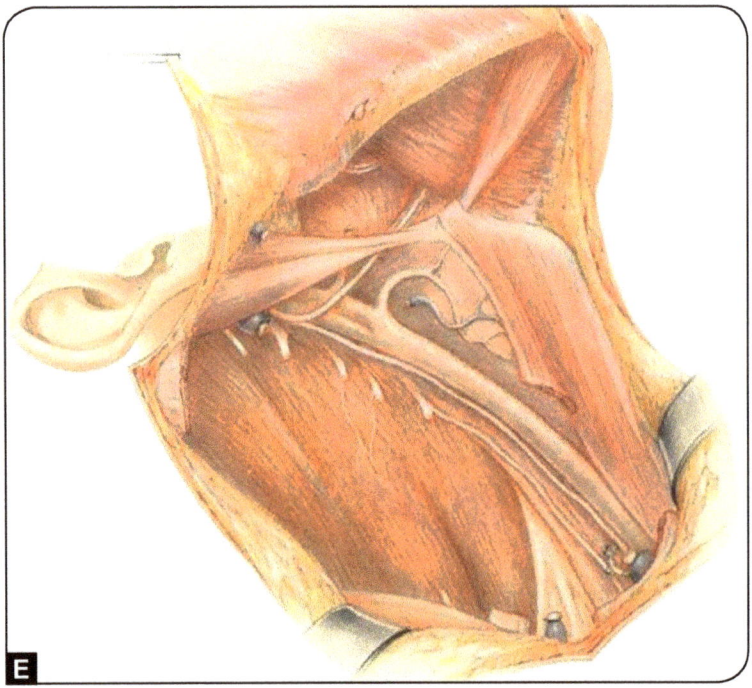

Fig. 6E

The incision is usually closed in two layers; the first one approximates the platysma anteriorly and the subcutaneous tissue laterally, and the second one approximates the skin. In general, it is best to avoid continuous suturing in the wound closure, since a seroma, a chyle collection, an abscess, or a pharyngocutaneous fistula may require the wound to be partially opened, postoperatively, for drainage.

One or two suction drains are left in place; they should not rest immediately over the carotid artery or in the area of the thoracic duct. Bulky or pressure dressings are unnecessary.

UNIQUE CONSIDERATIONS

Bilateral Radical Neck Dissection

In the occasional patient in whom a bilateral RND is necessary, the surgeon should alert the anesthesiologist to the possibility of resecting both IJVs. To avoid cerebral edema, which can in turn cause a syndrome of inappropriate secretion of ADH, fluid administration should be reduced to about 50 mL/hour after ligating the second IJV. In addition, it is often possible to preserve the external jugular vein in the least involved side of the neck, since this vein may be separated from the tumor by the SCMM and thus can be dissected free without compromising the cancer resection. Alternatively, a segment of saphenous vein can be used as a graft to replace one of the IJVs. In every case, serum and urine osmolality should be monitored to guide postoperative fluid replacement.

REFERENCES

1. Towpik E. First neck dissection. Gazeta Lekarska. 1888;85(3): 469.
2. Crile G. Excision of cancer of the head and neck. JAMA. 1906;47:1780-86.
3. Blair VP, Brown JB. The treatment of cancerous or potentially cancerous cervical lymph nodes. Ann Surg. 1933;98(4):650-61.
4. Martin H, Del Valle B, Ehrlich H, Cahan WG. Neck dissection. Cancer. 1951;4(3):441-99.
5. McQuarrie DG, Mayberg M, Ferguson M, Shons AR. A physiologic approach to the problems of simutaneous bilateral neck dissection. Am J Surg. 1977;134(4):455-60.

Modified Radical Neck Dissection with Preservation of the Spinal Accessory Nerve

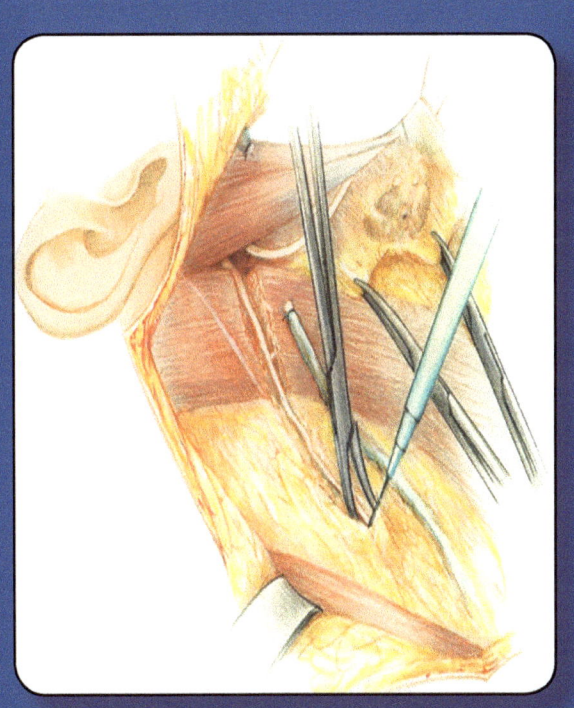

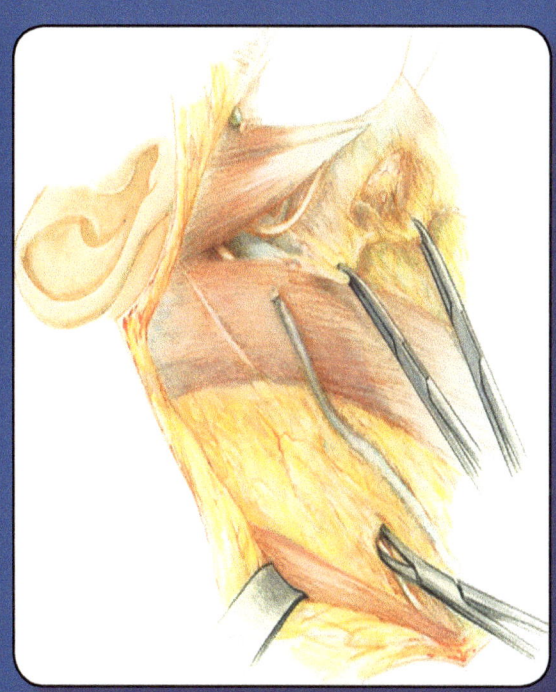

INTRODUCTION

This neck dissection consists of the removal of the lymph node bearing tissues of one side of the neck (levels I–V) preserving the spinal accessory nerve. Like in the radical neck dissection, the internal jugular vein (IJV) and the sternocleidomastoid muscle (SCMM) are included in the resected specimen.

The first descriptions of preservation of the spinal accessory nerve during a radical neck dissection date back to Dargent and Papillon[1] in 1945 and Ward and Robben[2] in 1951. More than three decades later, Saunders et al.[3] compared the resulting shoulder function in patients that underwent neck dissection with resection, preservation or reconstruction (cable graft) of the spinal accessory nerve. They found that symptoms related to shoulder dysfunction were mild or moderate in over 80% of the patients that had the nerve preserved or reconstructed with a cable graft. Since then, preservation of the spinal accessory nerve in the course of a radical neck dissection has been advocated on the basis of the following premises:

- First, in many instances, lymph nodes that are involved with tumor are not in immediate proximity to the spinal accessory nerve.
- Second, when a lymph node involved by tumor is close to the nerve, the nerve can be dissected and preserved, as it is commonly done with the facial nerve during parotid surgery.
- Third, and more importantly, preservation of the spinal accessory nerve, when appropriate, does not compromise the oncologic soundness of the operation.[4,5]
- Finally, the morbidity associated with the radical neck dissection, especially the shoulder pain and impairment of motion that results from resecting the spinal accessory nerve, can be quite disabling.

Thus, the desirability to preserve the nerve whenever is appropriate. It should be kept in mind, however, that preserving the spinal accessory nerve does not ensure adequate postoperative function of the trapezius. Moderate to severe electromyographic abnormalities and temporary dysfunction of the trapezius have been observed in patients that have undergone this operation.[6] Consequently, it is critical to handle the nerve carefully during surgery, avoiding undue traction and stretching of it.

INDICATIONS

Currently, the main role for this type of neck dissection is in the surgical treatment of the neck in selected patients with clinically obvious lymph node metastases, whenever the spinal accessory nerve is not directly involved by tumor, regardless of the number, size and location of the involved lymph nodes. Obviously then, the decision to preserve the spinal accessory nerve and, thus, the indication for this type of neck dissection is a delicate intraoperative judgment call. Much like the time-honored philosophy about preservation of the facial nerve during surgery for parotid tumors, the spinal accessory nerve can be preserved whenever there is a clearly identifiable, not an artificially created, plane of dissection between the tumor and the nerve.

SURGICAL TECHNIQUE

The incision to be used is chosen depending upon the factors described in Chapter 2.

Dissection of the Submandibular and Submental Triangles

It is performed as described in detail in sections 2A to 2J of Chapter 3.

Superior Lateral Dissection

Steps of superior lateral dissection are as follows:

- *1A:* This portion of the operation begins with the exposure of the posterior belly of the digastric, the upper most portion of the IJV, the spinal accessory nerve and the hypoglossal nerve. The technique to accomplish this safely is described in detail in Section 3A of Chapter 3.

- *1B:* With a hemostat used to elevate the portion of the SCMM that overlies the nerve, the muscle is divided obliquely down and backwards, exposing the portion of the nerve that courses through the muscle.

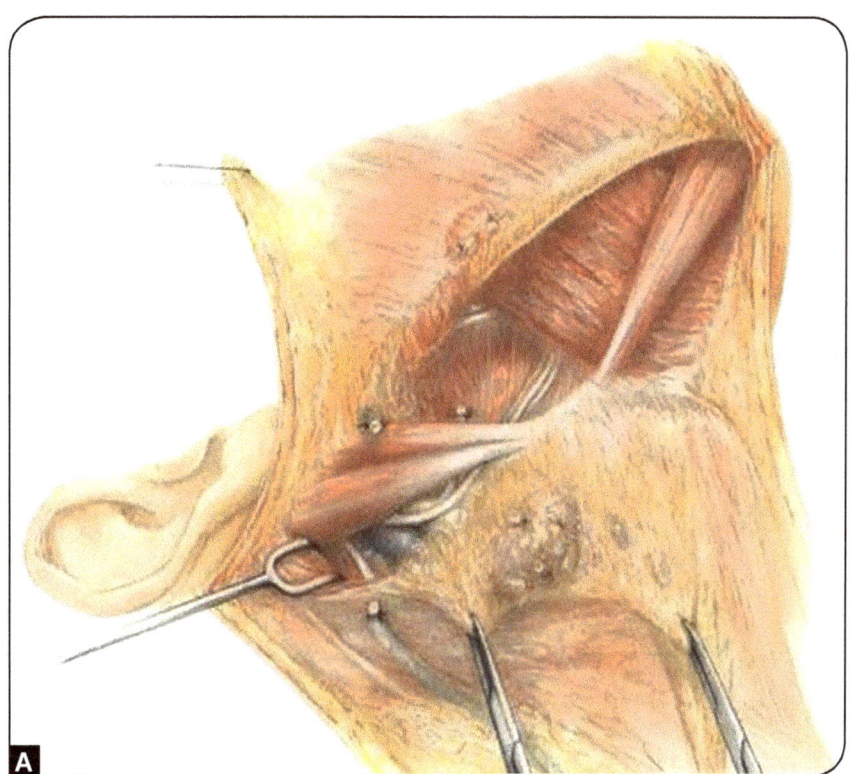

Fig. 1A

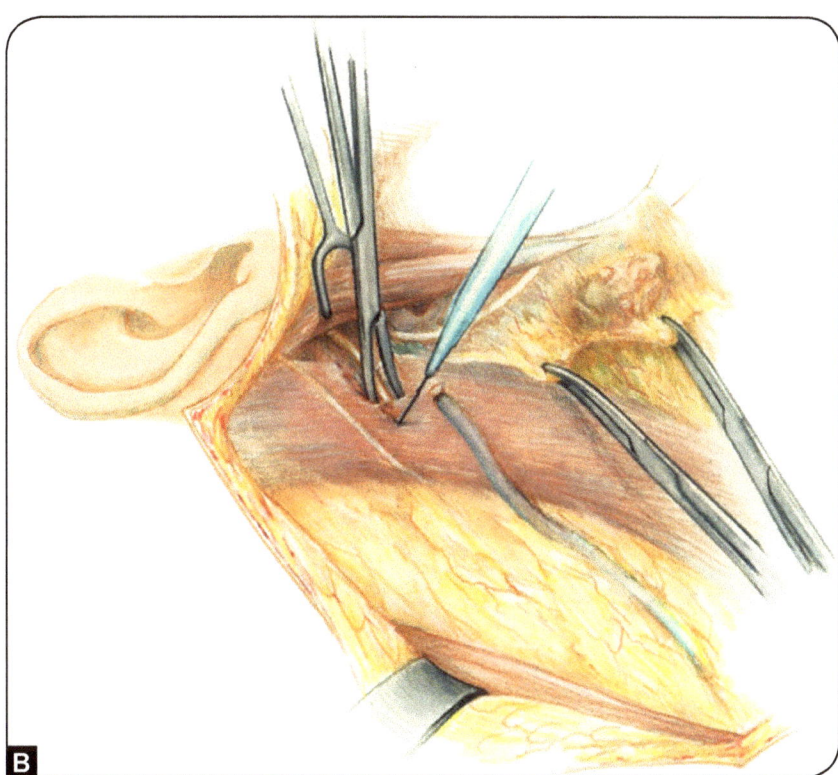

Fig. 1B

- *1C:* Using the same technique, the nerve is exposed through its course in the posterior triangle of the neck.

- *1D:* Alternatively, when it is not prudent to begin by exposing the nerve superiorly, the nerve is identified and initially exposed in front of the anterior border of the trapezius or in the mid-posterior triangle of the neck. From there, the nerve is followed in a cephalad direction and the SCMM is incised from below, upwards.

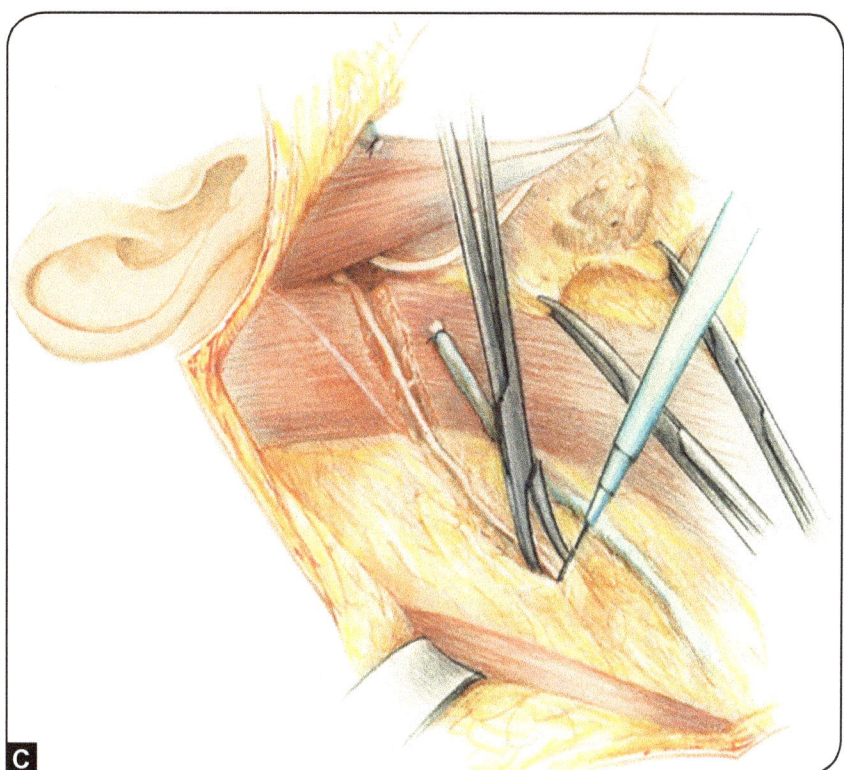

Fig. 1C

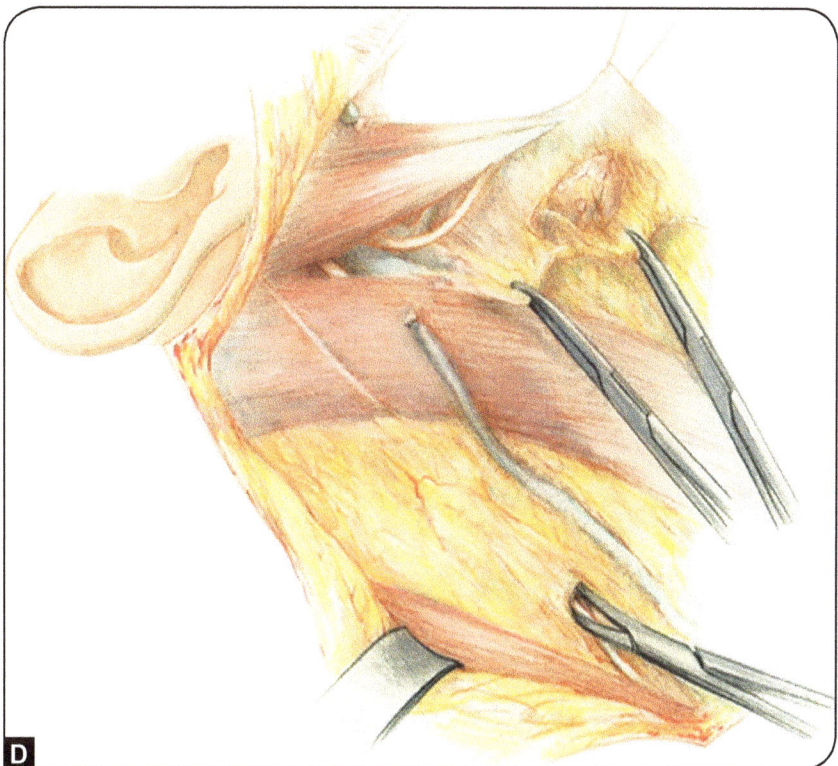

Fig. 1D

- *1E:* The branches of the spinal accessory nerve to the SCMM are divided leaving a short stump that can be grasped with a forceps or hemostat. This can then be used to exert gentle traction on the nerve to free it from the surrounding tissues, throughout its entire course in the neck.

- *1F:* The superior insertion of the SCMM is divided exposing the splenius capitis muscle posteriorly.

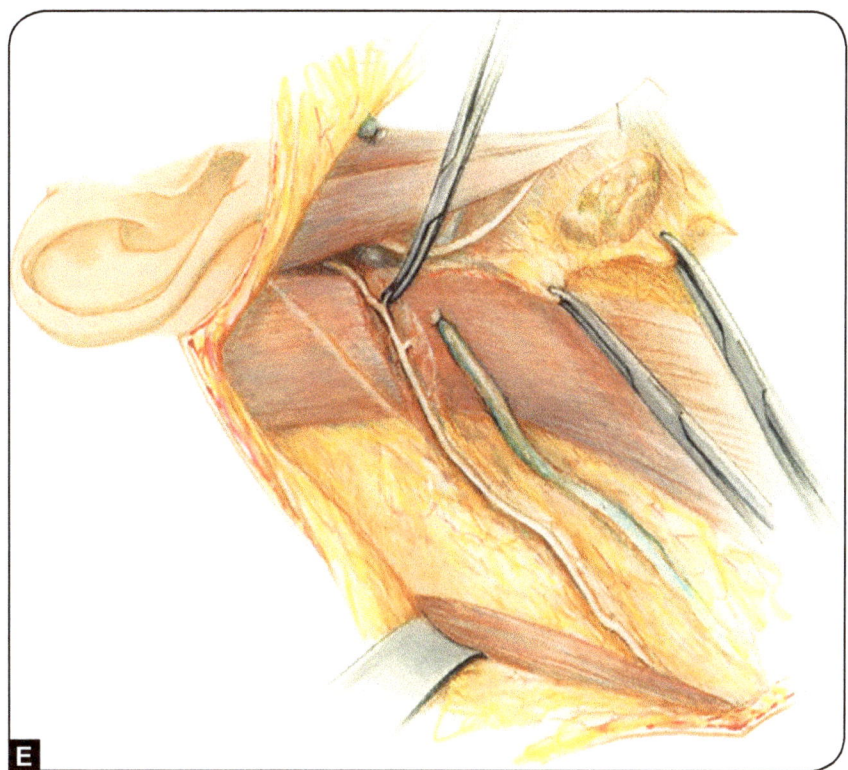

Fig. 1E

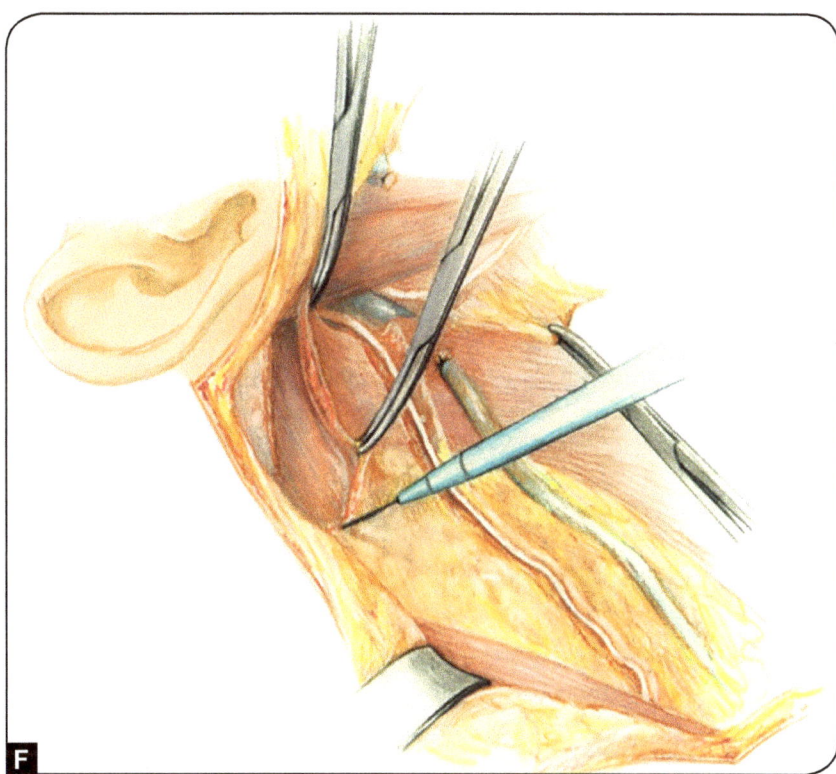

Figs. 1A to F: Superior lateral dissection.

Posterior Dissection

Steps of posterior dissection are as follows:

- *2A:* The dissection continues inferiorly, along the anterior border of the trapezius muscle and then forward over the splenius capitis muscle. These tissues are then brought forward under the spinal accessory nerve.

- *2B:* The dissection proceeds forward on to the levator scapula muscle. To preserve the nerves to the levator (arrow), the plane of dissection should be superficial to the fascia of it, provided that this does not compromise the adequacy of the resection of nodes involved by tumor. Further, superiorly, the upper most trunks of the cervical plexus are divided and, then, the upper end of the IJV is divided and doubly ligated.

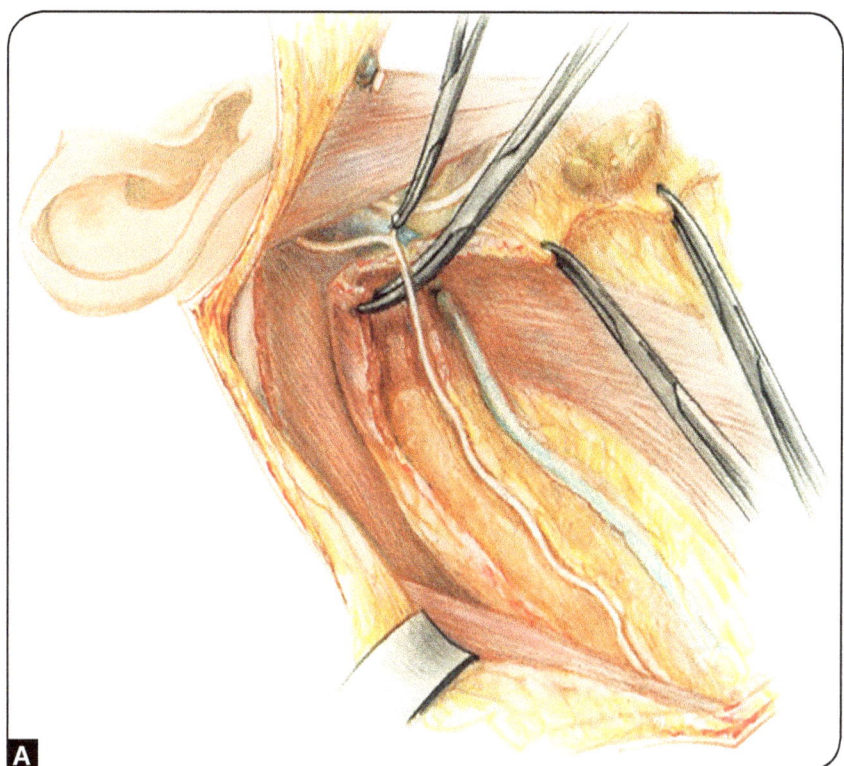

Fig. 2A

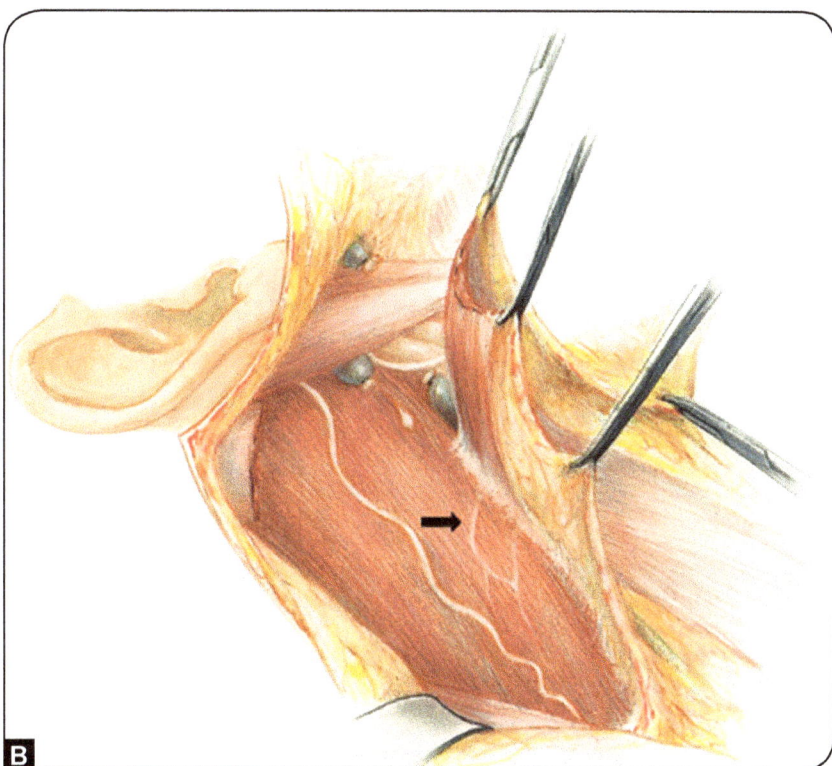

Fig. 2B

Inferior Dissection

Steps of inferior dissection are as follows:

- *3A:* Inferiorly, the lower insertion of the SCMM, the external jugular vein and the posterior belly of the omohyoid muscle are divided.

- *3B:* The fibro-fatty tissues above the clavicle are divided layer by layer exposing the brachial plexus and the phrenic nerve. For additional details about this portion of the operation, *see* Sections 5A to 5C in Chapter 3.

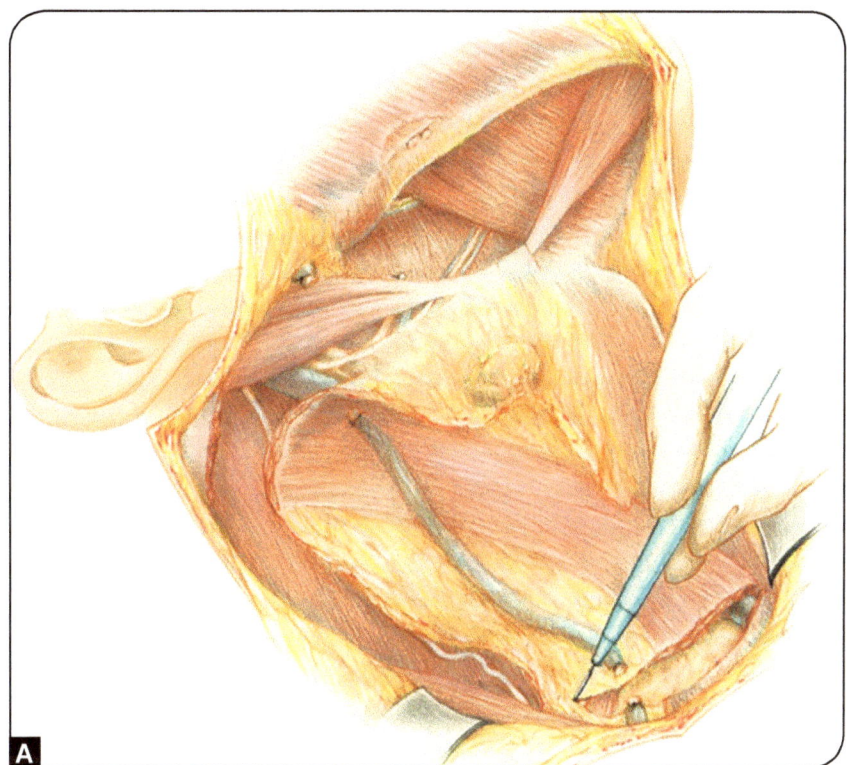

Fig. 3A

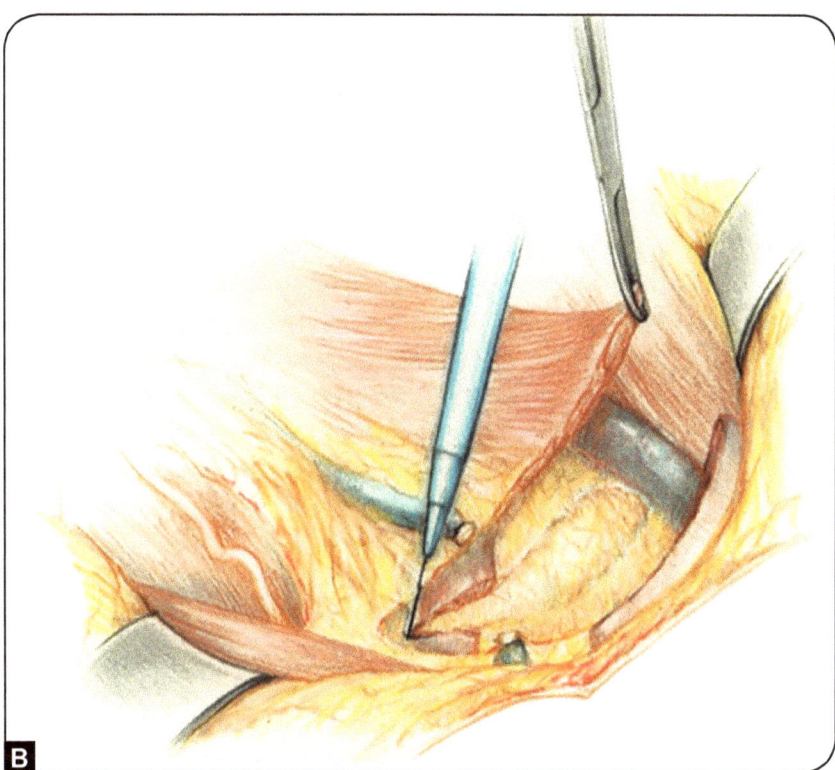

Figs. 3A and B: Inferior dissection.

Medial Dissection

Steps of medial dissection are as follows:

- *4A:* Medially and inferiorly, the thoracic duct (arrow), its afferents or both can be visualized and divided between clips. Then, the remaining trunks of the cervical plexus are divided and the inferior end of the IJV is divided and doubly ligated. For additional details about the anatomy of this area please see Figure 6B in Chapter 3.

- *4B:* The tissue between the IJV and the carotid and vagus nerve are sharply divided, including the anterior belly of the omohyoid muscle.

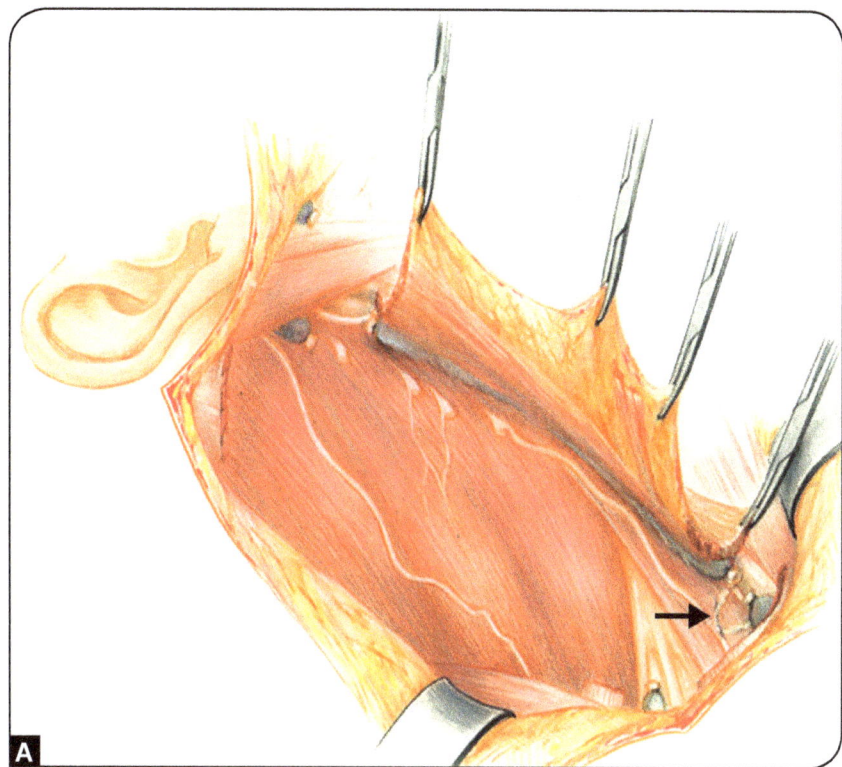

Fig. 4A

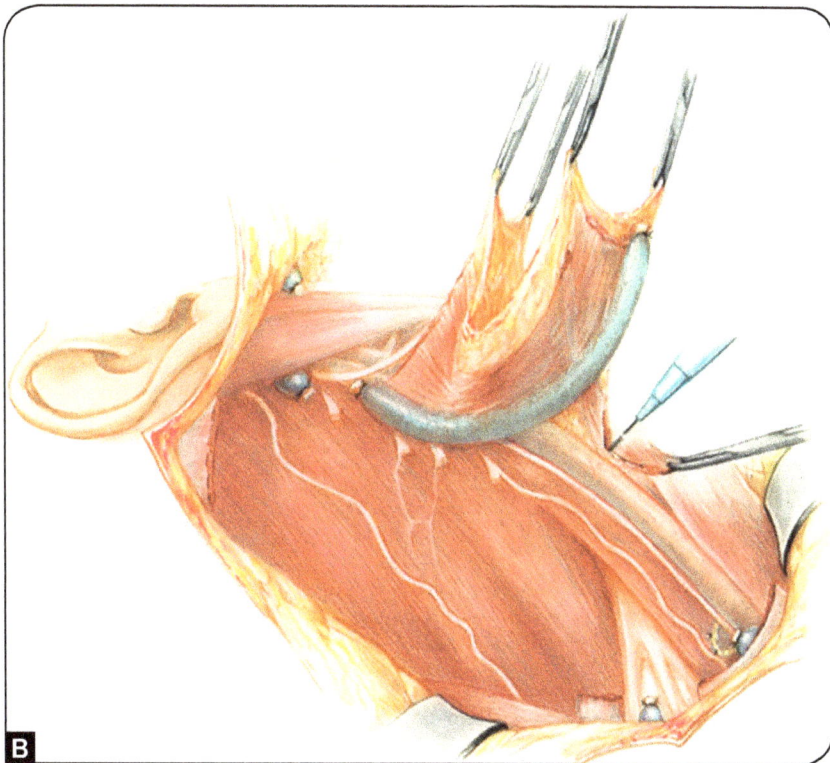

Fig. 4B

- *4C:* Finally, a thyro-lingual facial vein is divided with the hypoglossal nerve under direct vision to avoid accidentally injuring the nerve with the clamp.

- *4D:* Similar to the radical and other modified radical neck dissections, the completed dissection extends from the posterior belly of the digastric muscle superiorly to the clavicle inferiorly, and from the posterior border of the strap muscles anteriorly to the anterior border of the trapezius muscle.

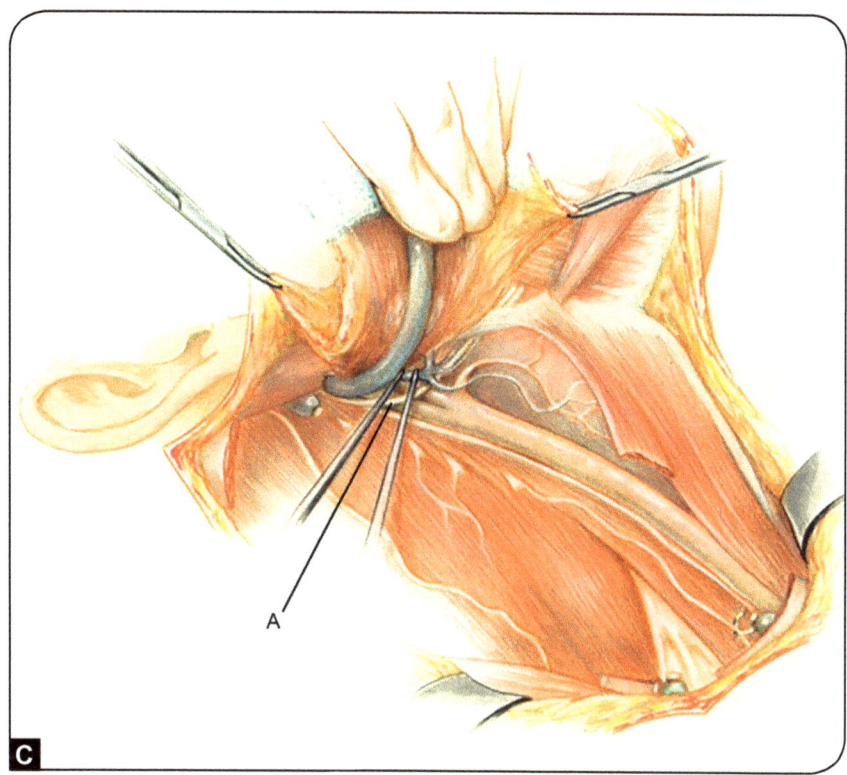

Fig. 4C: (A) Hypoglossal nerve.

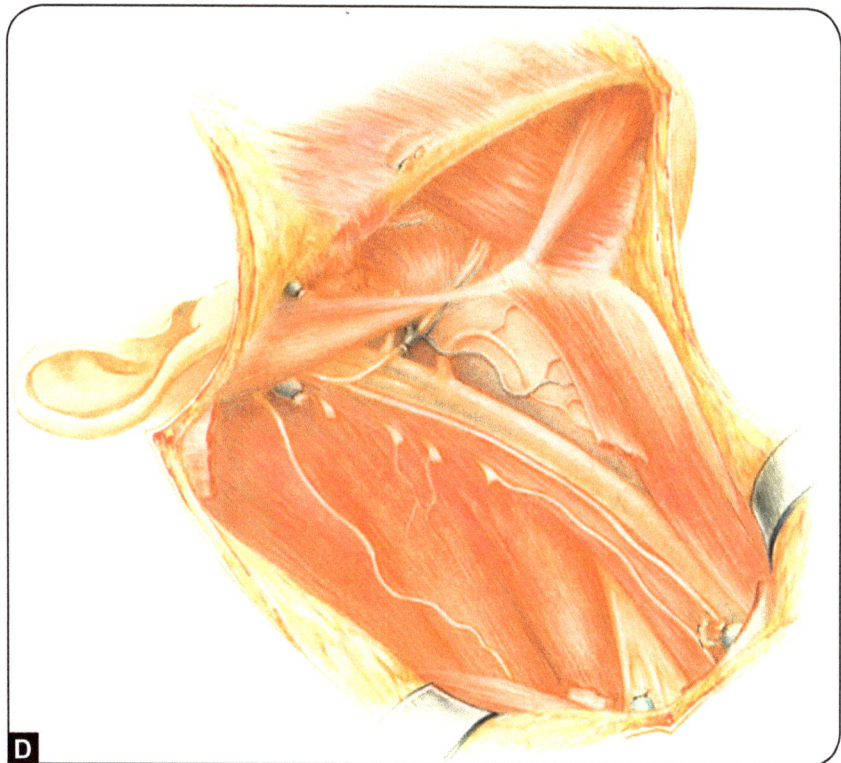

Fig. 4D: Completed dissection.

REFERENCES

1. Dargent M, Papillon J. Rersultats eloignes de lévididement ganglionnaire du cou avec conservation du filet mentonier et du spinal. Lyon Chir. 1945;41:715-22.
2. Ward GE, Robben JO. A composite operation for radical neck dissection and removal of cancer of the mouth. Cancer. 1951;4(1):98-109.
3. Saunders JR Jr, Hirata RM, Jaques DA. Considering the spinal accessory nerve in head and neck surgery. Am J Surg. 1985;150(4):491-94.
4. Skolnik EM, Tenta LT, Wineinger DM, et al. Preservation of XI cranial nerve in neck dissections. Laryngoscope. 1967;77(8): 1304-14.
5. Brandenburg JH, Lee CY. The eleventh nerve in radical neck surgery. Laryngoscope. 1981;91(11):1851-9.
6. Remmler D, Byers R, Scheetz J, et al. A prospective study of shoulder disability resulting from radical and modified neck dissections. Head Neck Surg. 1986;8(4):280-6.

CHAPTER 5

Modified Radical Neck Dissection with Preservation of the Spinal Accessory Nerve and the Internal Jugular Vein

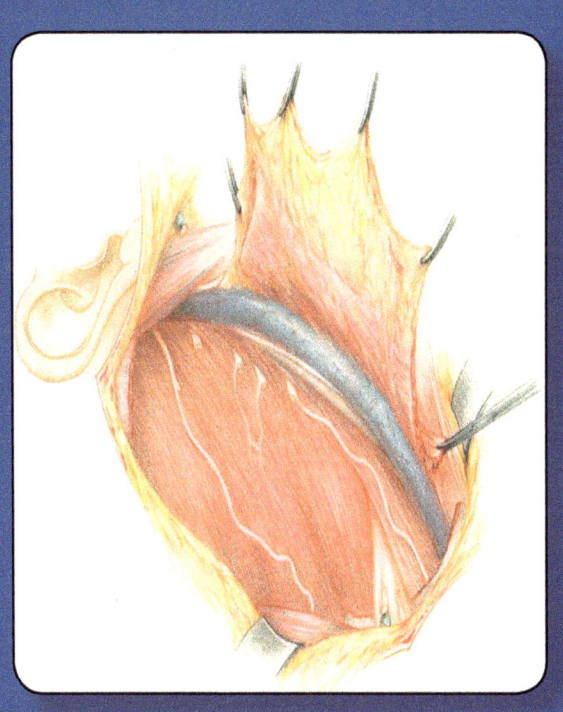
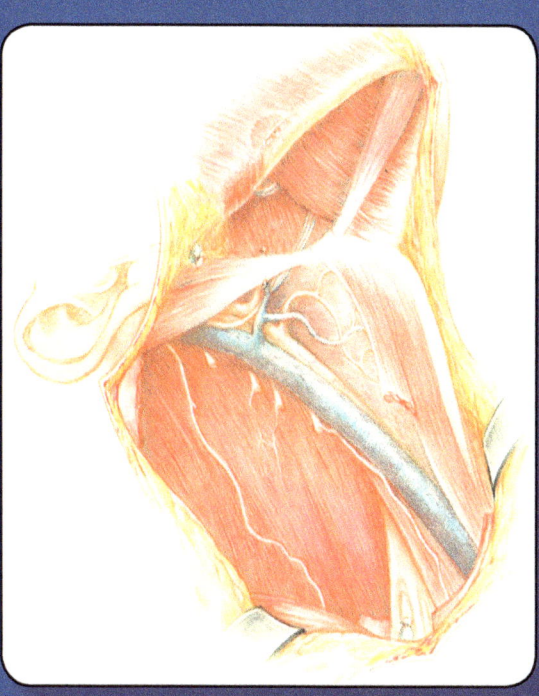

INTRODUCTION

This neck dissection consists of the removal of the lymph node bearing tissues of one side of the neck (levels I–V) preserving the spinal accessory nerve and the internal jugular vein (IJV). The sternocleidomastoid muscle (SCMM) is included in the resected specimen.

INDICATIONS

The decision to preserve the spinal accessory nerve and the IJV is made by the surgeon intraoperatively. The spinal accessory nerve can be preserved whenever there is a clearly identifiable, not an artificially created, plane of dissection between the tumor and the nerve. The IJV can be preserved occasionally in the presence of metastases at different levels of the neck, particularly in some cases of metastatic papillary thyroid cancer and, less often, melanoma. Metastases from these tumors, unlike most squamous cell carcinomas, may grow in a more pushing and less infiltrative manner, making preservation of the vein possible. When dissecting lymph nodes off of the IJV, any change in the appearance, colour or thickness of the vein, usually apparent as a whitish discolouration of it (Fig. 1), should alert the surgeon about tumor involvement of the vein wall and prompt its removal.

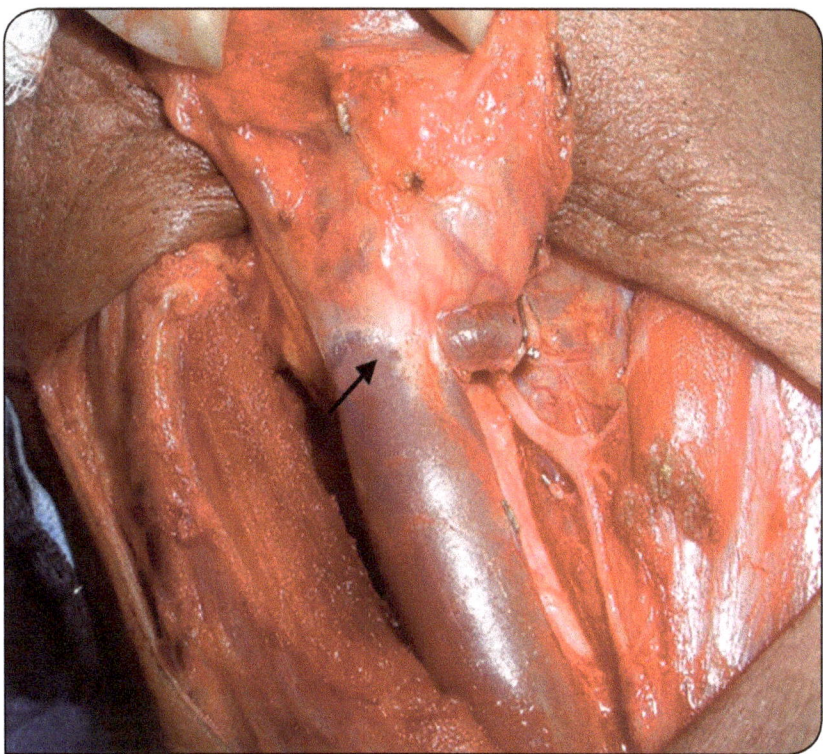

Fig. 1: Arrow points to area where proximity of tumor causes the wall of the vein to appear whitish and thicker.

SURGICAL TECHNIQUE

The incision to be used is chosen depending upon the factors described in Chapter 2.

Dissection of the Submandibular and Submental Triangles

It is performed as described in detail in Sections 2A to 2J of Chapter 3.

Superior Lateral, Posterior and Inferior Portions of the Dissection

These are performed as described for the modified radical neck dissection (MRND) with preservation of the spinal accessory nerve in Sections 1, 2 and 3 of Chapter 4.

Medial Dissection

Steps of medial dissection are as follows:

- *2A:* The specimen is rotated forward exposing the posterior and lateral aspects of the IJV.

- *2B:* The fibro-fatty tissue and lymph nodes adjacent to the anterior and anterior-medial aspects of the vein are dissected sharply; the anterior belly of the omohyoid muscle is divided.

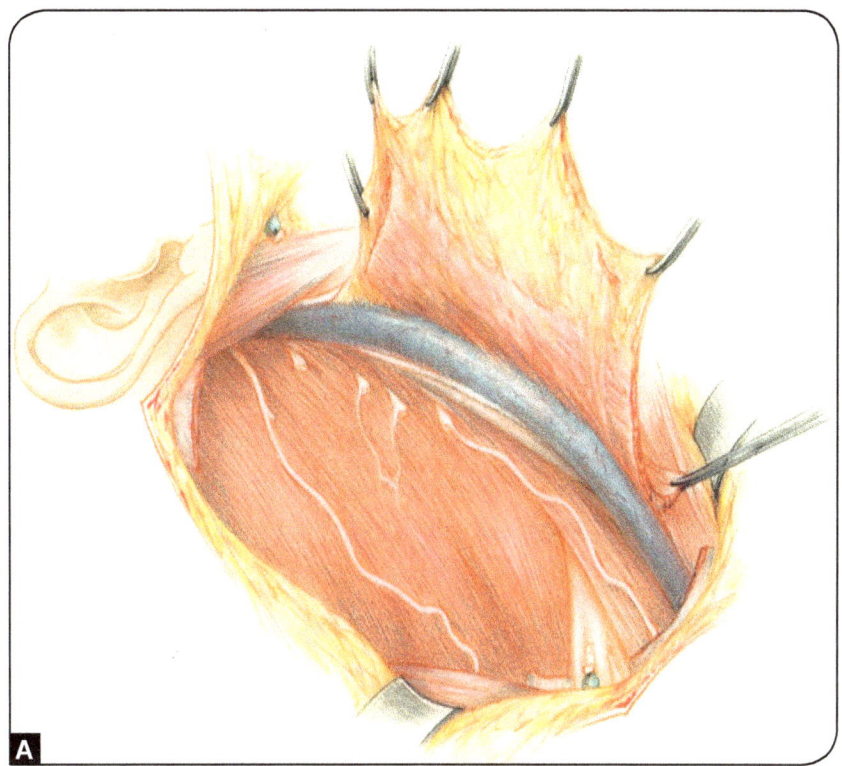

Fig. 2A

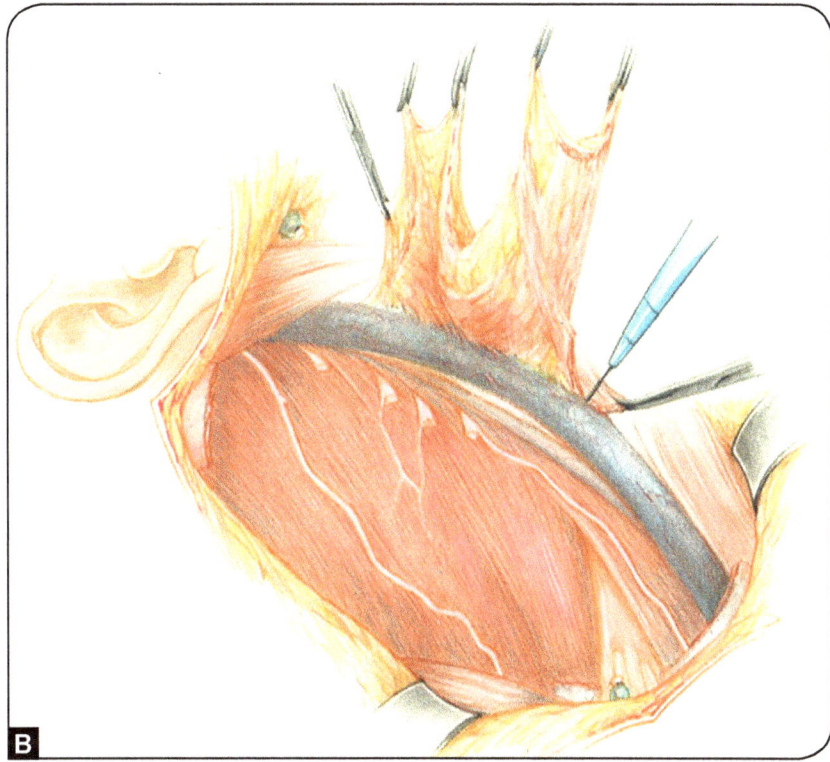

Fig. 2B

- *2C:* The anterior facial vein is divided and ligated lateral to the plane of the hypoglossal nerve, which is kept under vision to prevent injuring it.

- *2D:* Like the radical and other MRNDs, the completed dissection extends from the posterior belly of the digastric muscle superiorly to the clavicle inferiorly, and from the posterior border of the strap muscles anteriorly to the anterior border of the trapezius muscle.

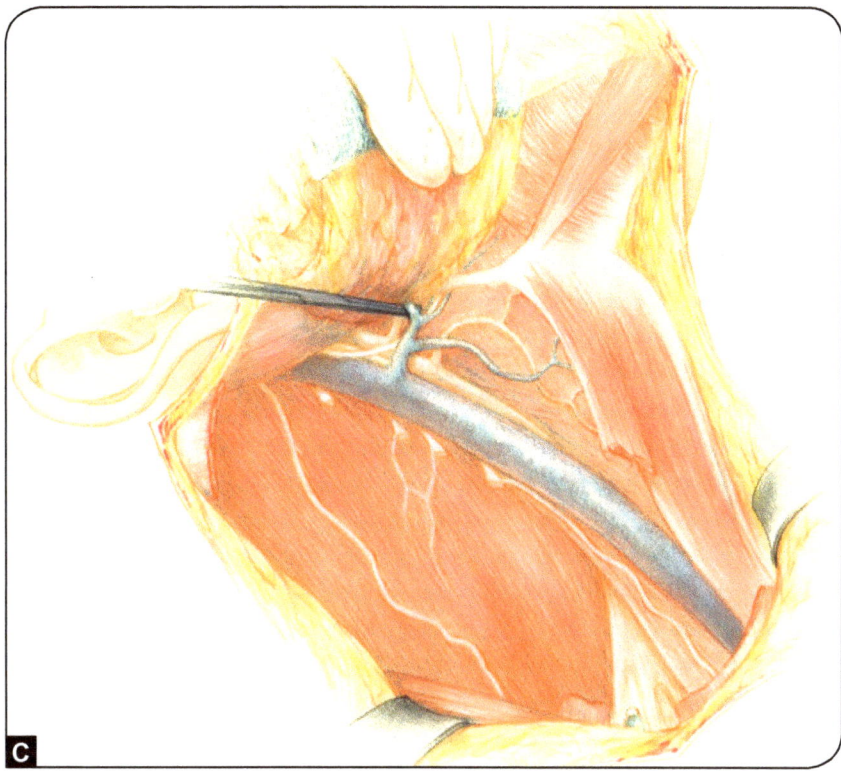

Fig. 2C

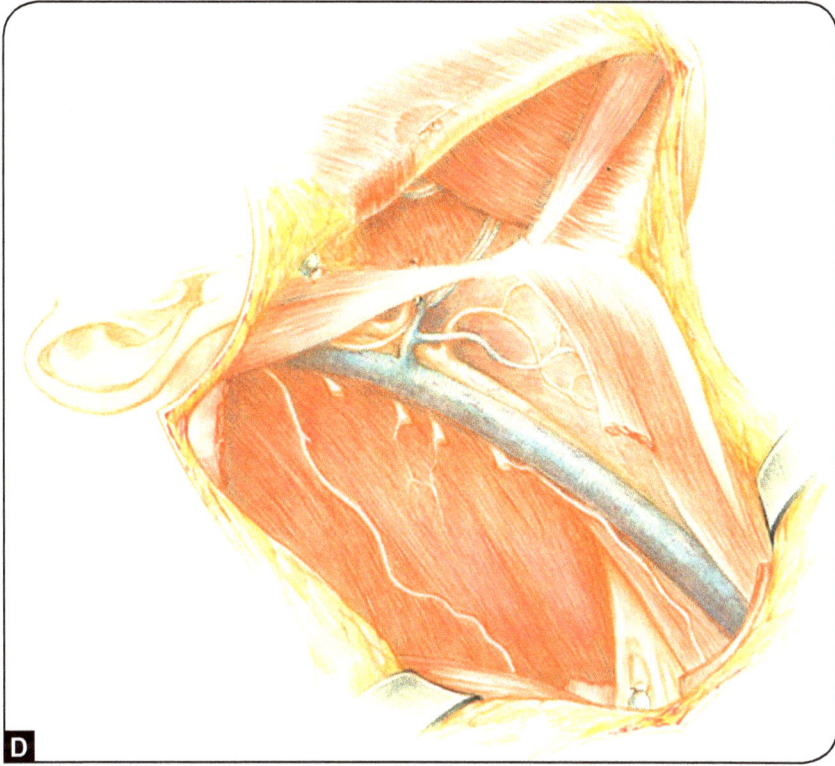

Fig. 2D: Completed MRND with preservation of the IJV and XIN.

CHAPTER 6

Modified Radical Neck Dissection Preserving the Spinal Accessory Nerve, the Internal Jugular Vein and the Sternocleidomastoid Muscle

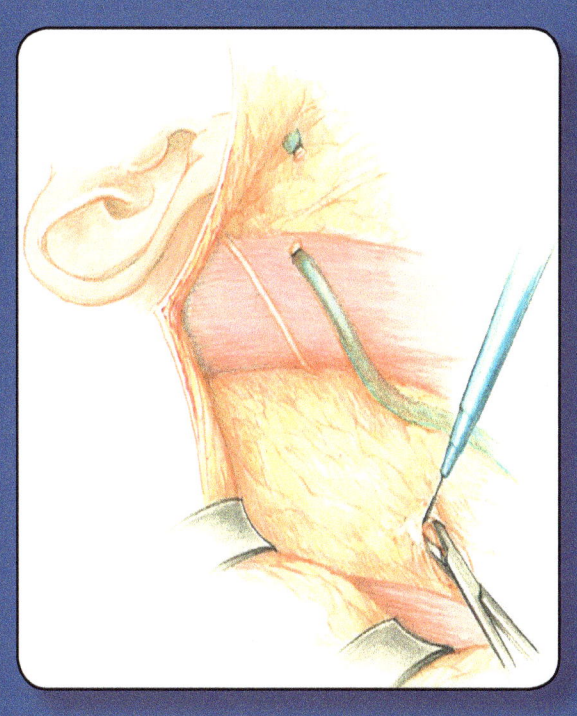
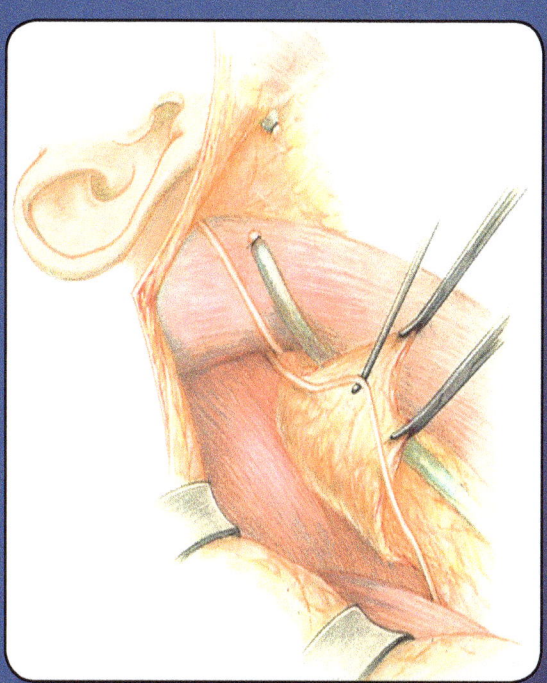

INTRODUCTION

This operation consists of the en block removal of the lymph node-bearing tissues of one side of the neck, including lymph nodes levels II–V, preserving the spinal accessory nerve, the internal jugular vein (IJV) and the sternocleidomastoid muscle (SCMM). The submandibular and submental triangles may or may not be included in the dissection.

The concept of removing "completely the lymph node containing tissues of the neck in conjunction with the primary and respecting noble structures" was substantiated by Osvaldo Suarez in 1963[1,2] with his observations in autopsy and surgery specimens of patients with cancer of the larynx and hypopharynx. He described a surgical technique and called it "functional dissection" as it "eliminates all the areolar tissue, fascia and lymph nodes and leaves the muscles, great vessels and noble parts without mutilation". In 1954 in Poland, Miodonski[3] had reported his experience with the same concept. It was, Bocca, however, who later popularized this operation, introduced the terms conservative and conservation neck dissection to designate it, emphasized that the muscular and vascular aponeurosis of the neck define compartments filled with fibroadipose tissue and that the lymphatic system of the neck, contained within these compartments, can be excised in an anatomic block by stripping the fascia off of muscles and vessels.[4,5]

This operation was advocated by many, particularly in Europe, as the neck dissection of choice for the treatment of the N0 neck in patients with squamous cell carcinoma of the upper aerodigestive tract, especially when the primary tumor is located in the larynx and hypopharynx. In that case, the nodes in the submandibular triangle are at low risk of containing metastases and do not need to be removed. Several surgeons advocated this operation also for the treatment of the neck in stage N1, when the metastatic nodes are mobile and no greater than 2.5–3 cm.[6-8] Bocca et al.[9] on the other hand, believed that the indications for this type of modified radical neck dissection are the same as those of the radical neck dissection and that the only contraindication to its use is the presence of node fixation.

Currently, this type of neck dissection is the operation of choice for patients with differentiated carcinoma of the thyroid gland who have palpable lymph node metastases in the lateral and posterior compartments of the neck.

SURGICAL TECHNIQUE

The position of the patient on the operating table and the surgical incisions are similar to those recommended for the radical neck dissection. The elevation of the cervical flaps and, if necessary, the dissection of the submental and submandibular triangles are performed in the manner described for the radical neck dissection. As the posterior skin flap is elevated, it should be kept in mind that the spinal accessory nerve is rather superficially located in the mid-posterior triangle of the neck, and it can be injured during this step of the operation. By the same token, during the elevation of this flap, the superficially located nerve is often stimulated by the electric cautery, giving the surgeon a hint as to the location of the nerve.

Once the flaps are elevated, depending upon the preference of the surgeon, the dissection may begin in the posterior triangle of the neck, or it may begin superiorly, especially if the submandibular triangle has been dissected. In this description, we will begin the dissection posteriorly.

Dissection of the Spinal Accessory Nerve in the Posterior Triangle of the Neck

Steps of dissection of the spinal accessory nerve in the posterior triangle of the neck are as follows:

- *1A*: The dissection of the posterior triangle begins by identifying the spinal accessory nerve. This can be done where the nerve crosses the anterior border of the trapezius muscle. However, exposure of the nerve in this area may be hampered by its proximity to the transverse cervical artery and to one or more veins. Using a mosquito type hemostat, a thin layer of fat or fascial tissue is elevated and incised in a direction perpendicular to the nerve. This maneuver is repeated until the nerve is clearly seen (Figure inset). Then, using the hemostat parallel to and immediately above the nerve, the tissues overlying it are incised, exposing the nerve in a cephalad direction.

- *1B*: The nerve can also be identified at the point where it exits from under the SCMM, a point usually located within 1 cm above Erb's point; once again, this may not the best area to expose the nerve initially, since here the nerve is located deep within the fibrofatty tissue posterior to the SCMM; furthermore, it can be confused with upper branches of the cervical plexus, which are parallel and slightly deep to it. If the nerve is exposed here, it is then freed from the surrounding tissues in a caudal direction.

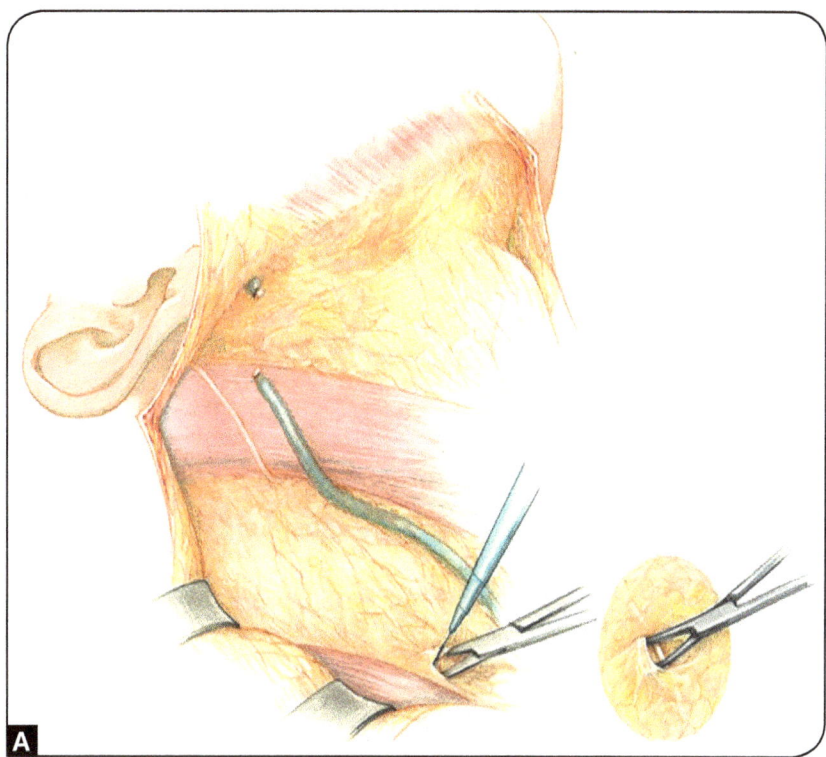

Fig. 1A

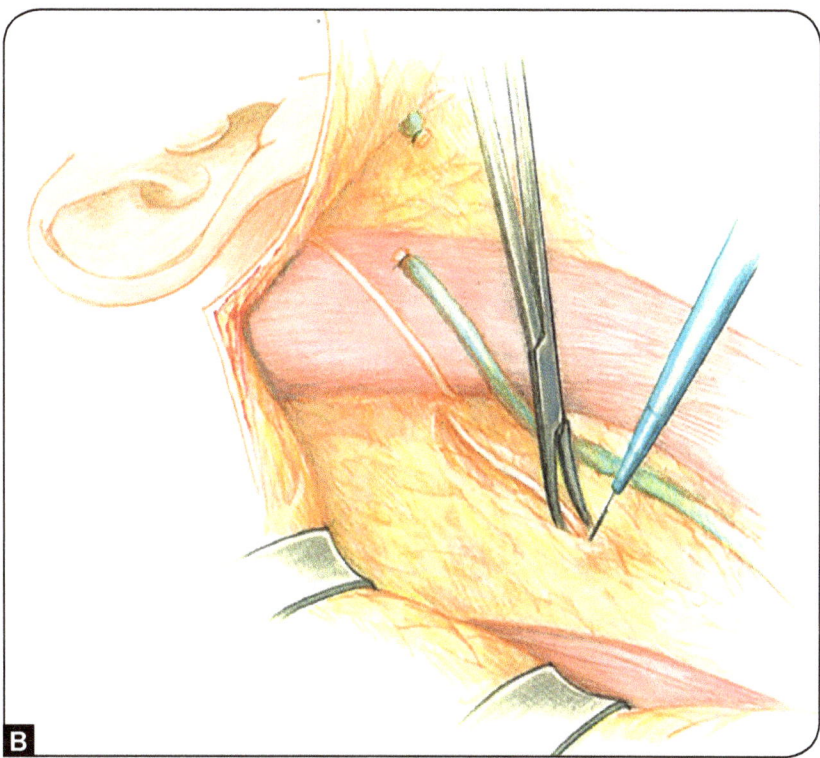

Fig. 1B

- *1C*: The nerve is more easily identified and exposed, as it courses in an oblique direction through the midportion of the posterior triangle of the neck, where it is more superficial. Oftentimes, it can be seen as the posterior skin flap is elevated. Once the nerve is clearly seen, using the hemostat parallel to and immediately above the nerve, the tissues overlying it are incised, exposing the nerve through the entire posterior triangle. Keep in mind that, in this area of the neck, the nerve usually has a curling course; thus, applying gentle traction on the nerve to straighten it facilitates its dissection.

- *1D:* Applying very gentle retraction on the nerve, a scalpel is used to free the nerve from the surrounding tissues throughout its entire course in the posterior triangle of the neck.

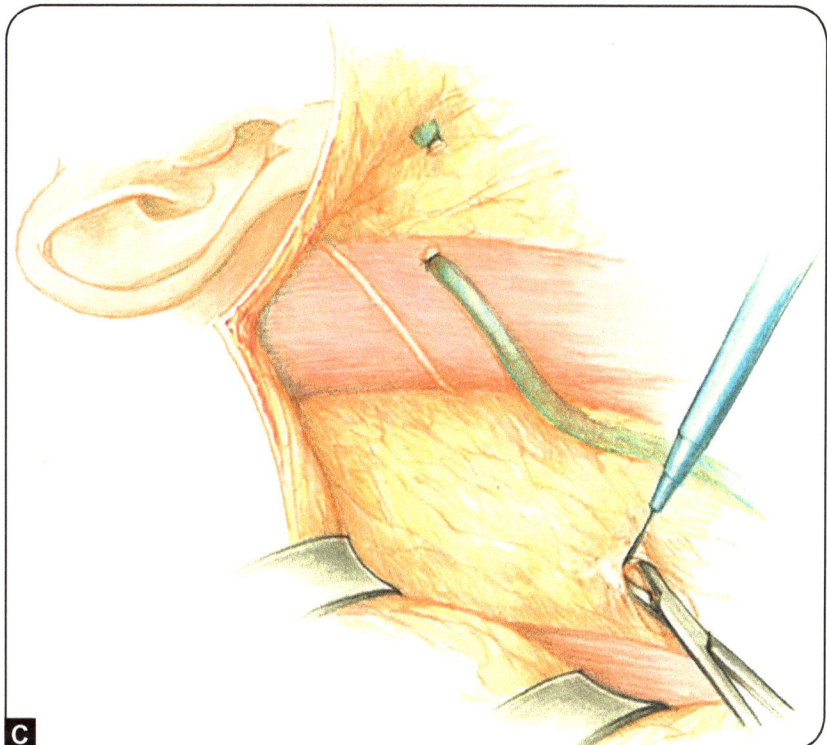

Fig. 1C

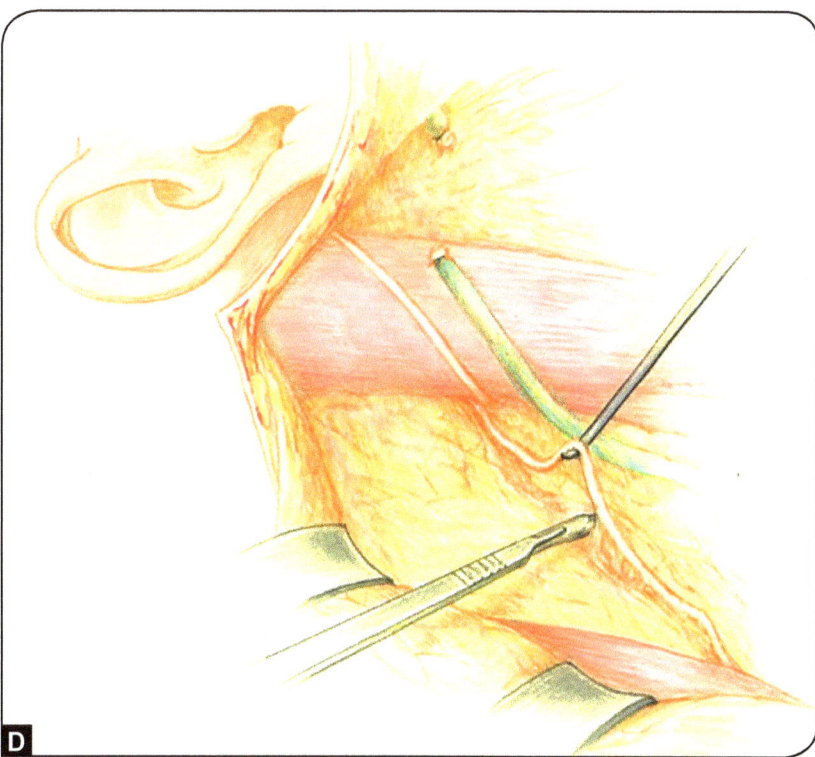

Fig. 1D

Dissection of the Posterior Triangle

Steps of dissection of the posterior triangle are as follows:

- *1E*: With the nerve isolated, the fascia and fibroadipose tissues are incised along the anterior border of the trapezius muscle. These tissues become thinner superiorly, where it is easier to reach and expose the splenius capitis muscle.

- *1F*: The fibro-fatty tissue that contains lymph nodes is then dissected in an anterior and inferior direction off of the splenius capitis and the levator scapulae muscles. The fascia of the splenius is very thin and the dissection is carried immediately over the muscle.

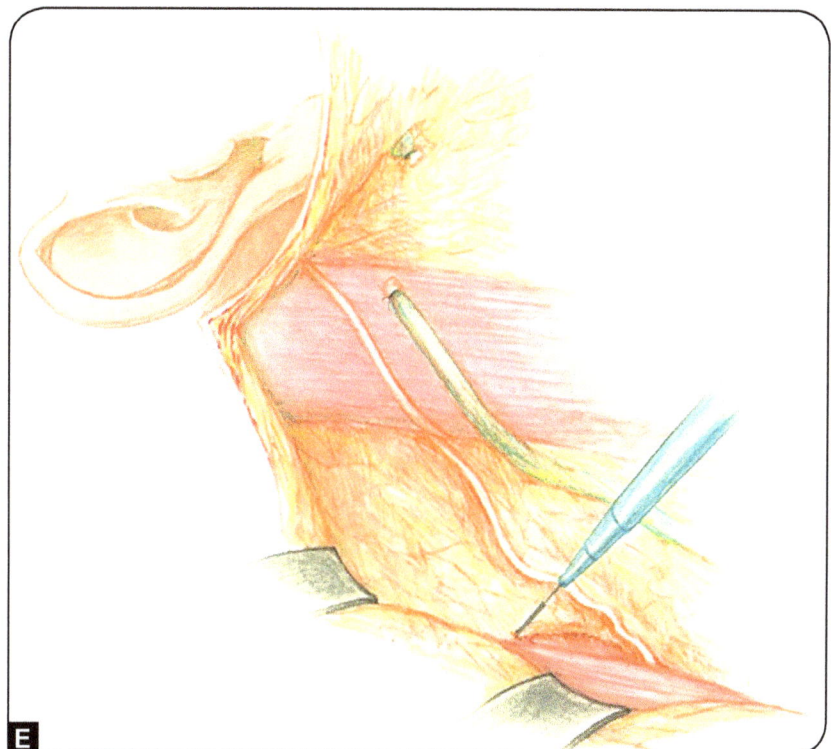

Fig. 1E

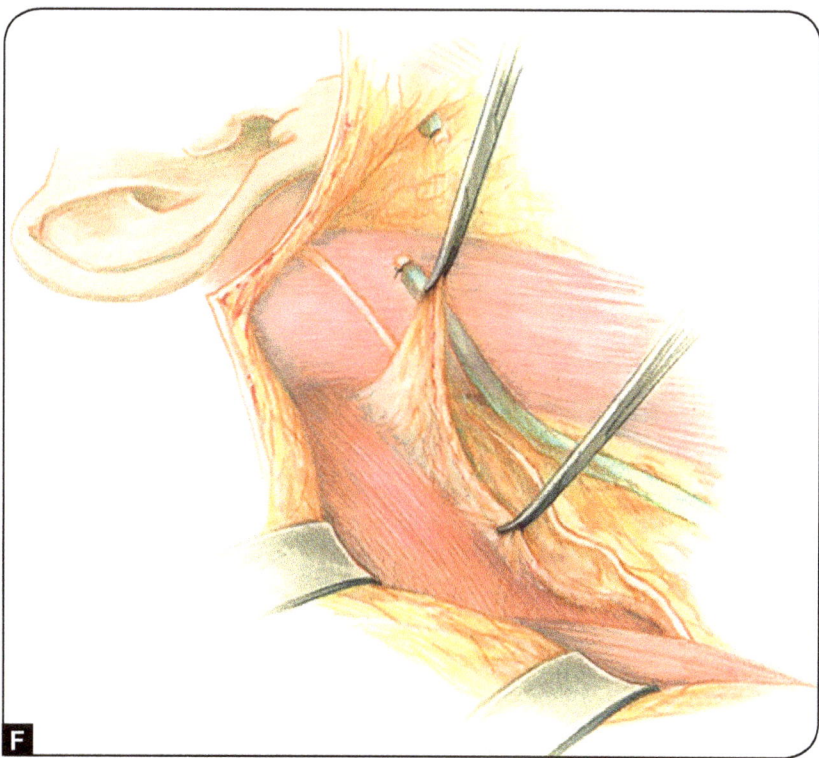

Fig. 1F

- *1G*: The specimen is then brought forward under the spinal accessory nerve.

- *1H*: As the dissection progresses on to the levator scapulae, an effort must be made to remain superficial to the fascia of the muscle in order to preserve the nerves to it, which lie immediately below its relatively thin fascia.

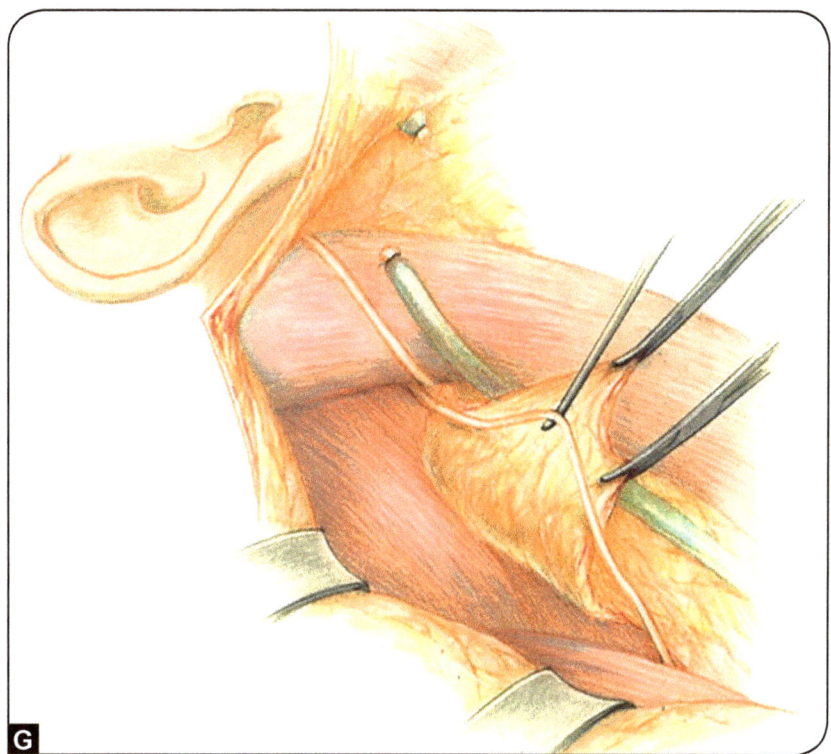

Fig. 1G

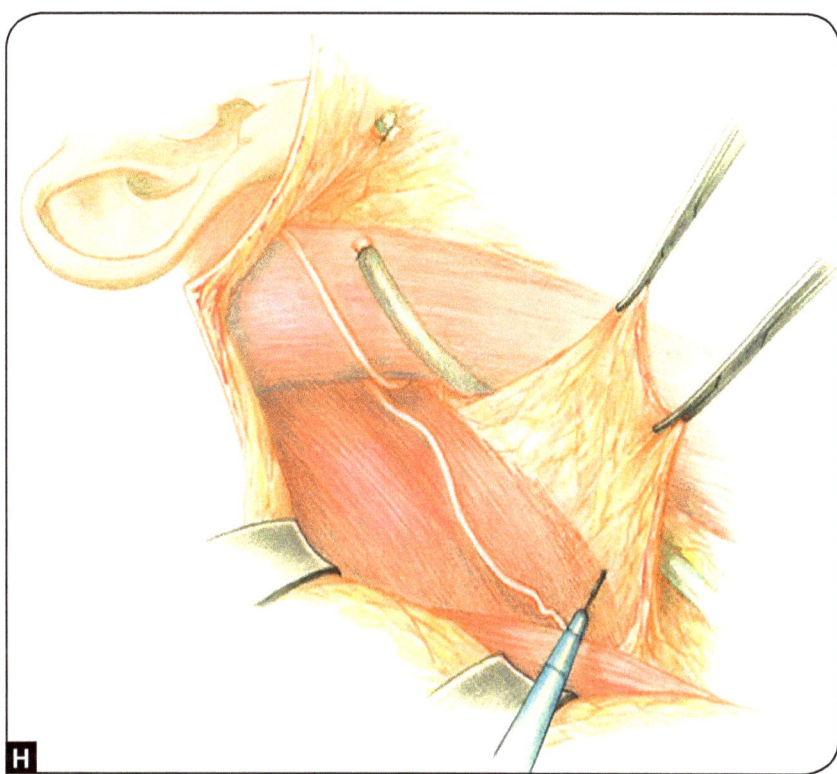

Fig. 1H

- *1I*: The fascia of the SCMM is incised along the lateral aspect and posterior border of the muscle. In doing this, the upper end of the external jugular vein is divided and the vein is dissected with the fascia. However, in many instances, the greater auricular nerve can be preserved.

- *1J*: The fascia is dissected off of the muscle in a circumferential manner, posteriorly and then off the medial aspect of the muscle, until the anterior border of it is reached; at that point, the shadow of the IJV may be seen anteriorly (arrow).

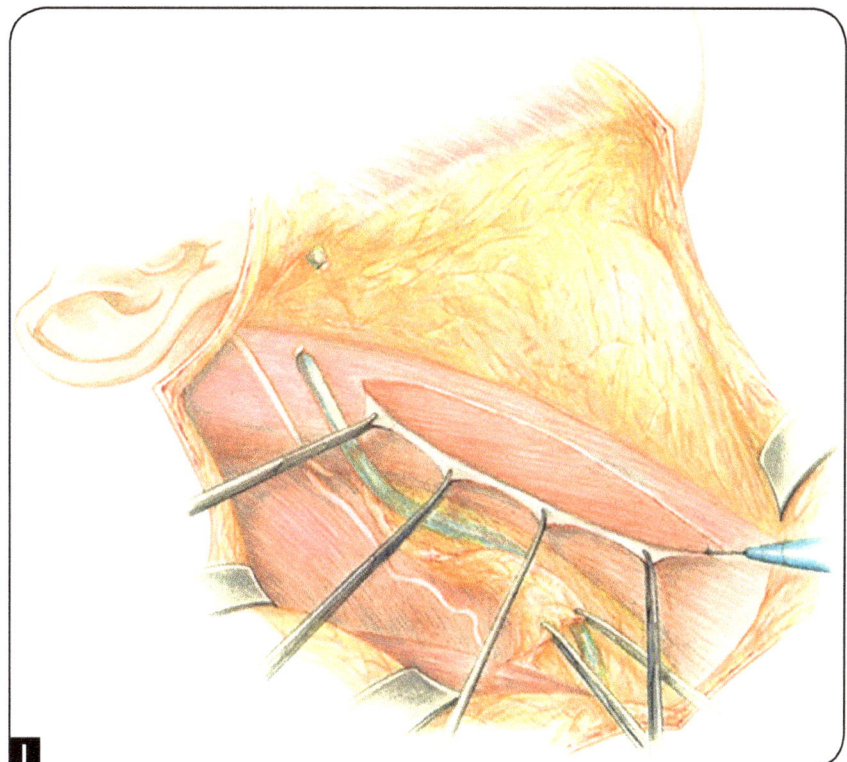

Fig. 1I

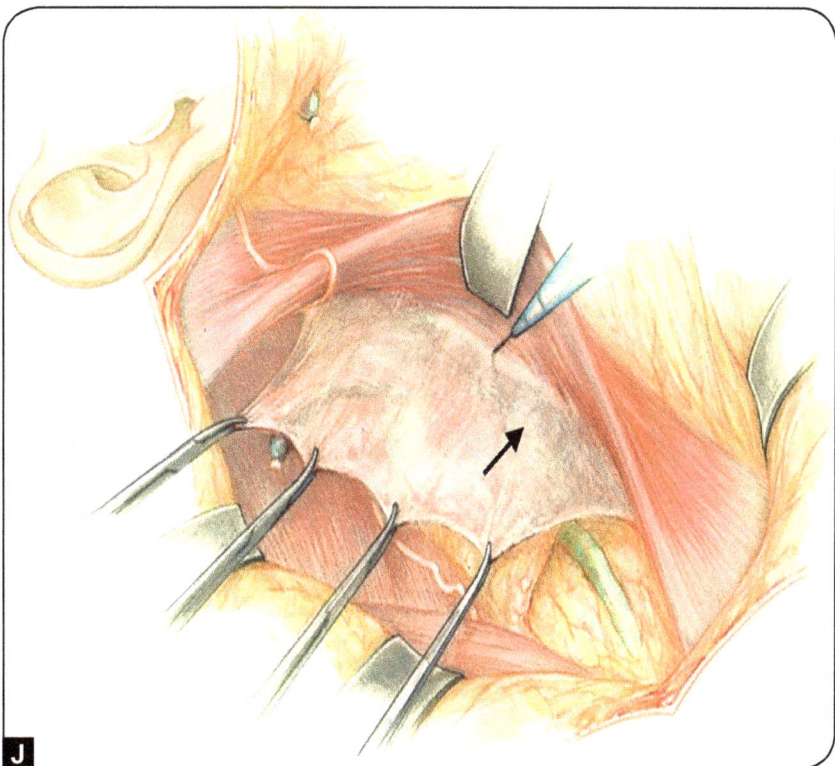

Fig. 1J

- *1K*: Retracting the inferior portion of the SCMM, the supraclavicular area is exposed between the shadow of the IJV and the anterior border of the trapezius. The inferior end of the external jugular vein is divided and ligated. Then, the superficial layer of the deep cervical fascia and several layers of fascia-like tissue are incised, as is the posterior belly of the omohyoid muscle. The cutaneous branches of the cervical plexus are also divided immediately above the clavicle.

- *1L*: The tissues in the supraclavicular area can then be swept in an upward direction, identifying the proper plane of dissection, superficial to the fascia of the scalenus muscles, the brachial plexus and the phrenic nerve. Care is taken to visualize and cauterize, or preferably clip or ligate small branches of the transverse cervical vessels coming toward the specimen.

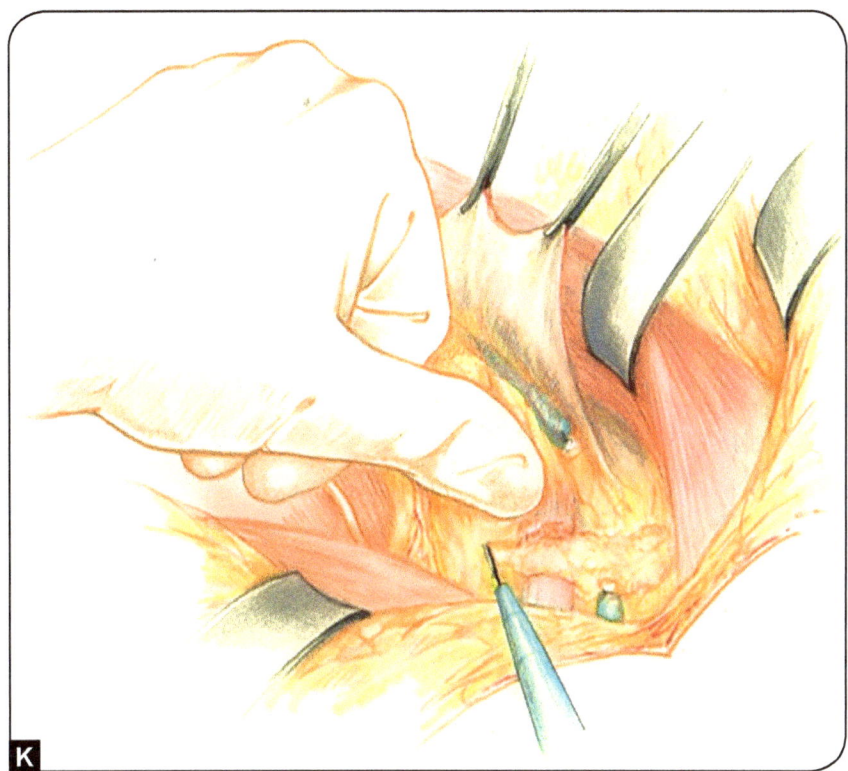

Fig. 1K

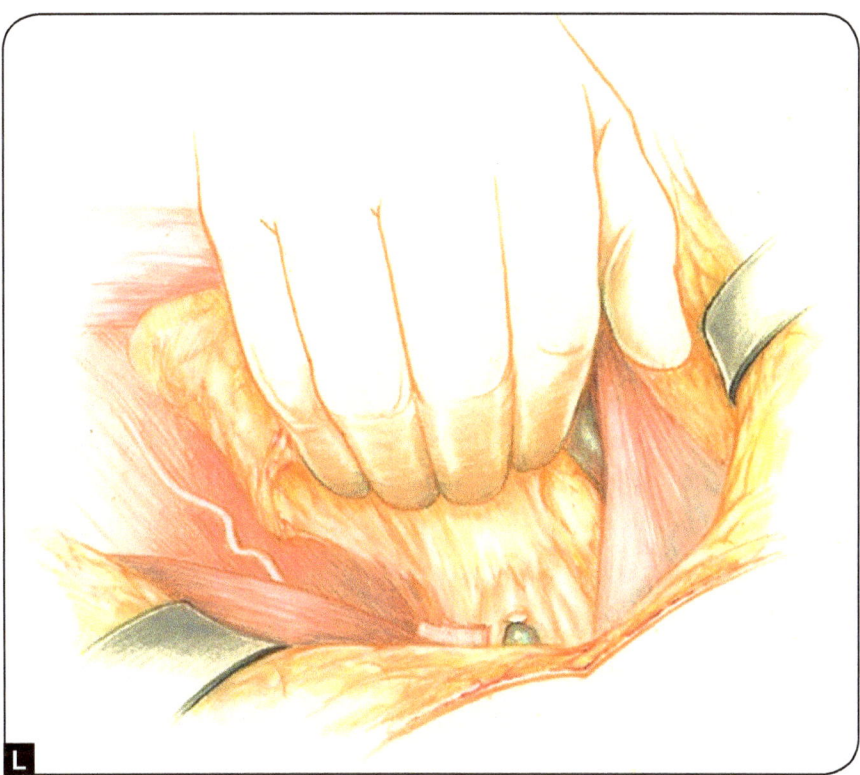

Fig. 1L

■   *1M*: The contents of the posterior triangle of the neck are now completely freed.

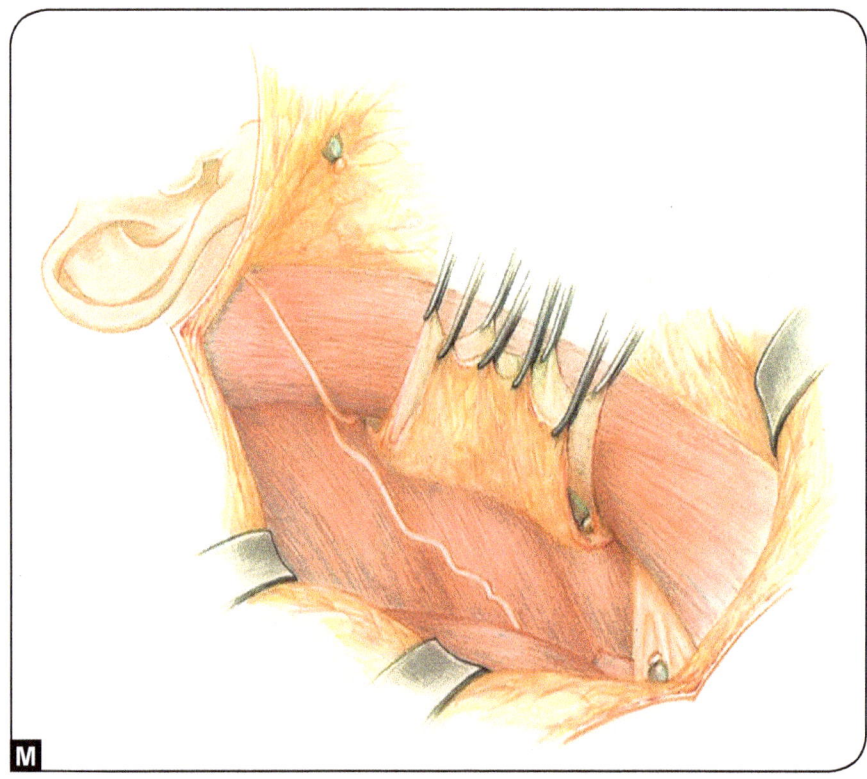

Fig. 1M

Superior and Lateral Dissection

The tissues immediately below and behind the submandibular gland are incised in several layers until the posterior belly of the digastric muscle is exposed. As in other neck dissections, depending upon the location and the extent of the tumor in the neck, the tail of the parotid gland may be dissected and retracted superiorly or transected, if necessary, to provide an adequate tissue margin above a large or a high level II (jugulodigastric) node involved with tumor. Likewise, it may be necessary to include the posterior belly of the digastric in the dissected specimen.

Steps of superior and lateral dissection are as follows:

- *2A*: The posterior belly of the digastric is slightly retracted upwards with an Army-Navy or a similar retractor. Then, with careful dissection, the upper most portion of the IJV, the spinal accessory nerve and the hypoglossal nerve are exposed. A useful technique to accomplish this safely consists of applying gentle inferior traction to the "specimen" and using a fine tip hemostat, such as a mosquito clamp, a thin layer of tissue is pierced; then, changing the angle of the clamp, as needed, the tip of the clamp is gently driven forward, under a thin layer of fascia or tissue. Opening the clamp a few millimeters, and elevating with it a "see-through" layer of tissue, allows the surgeon to cut the tissues without injuring the underlying structures.

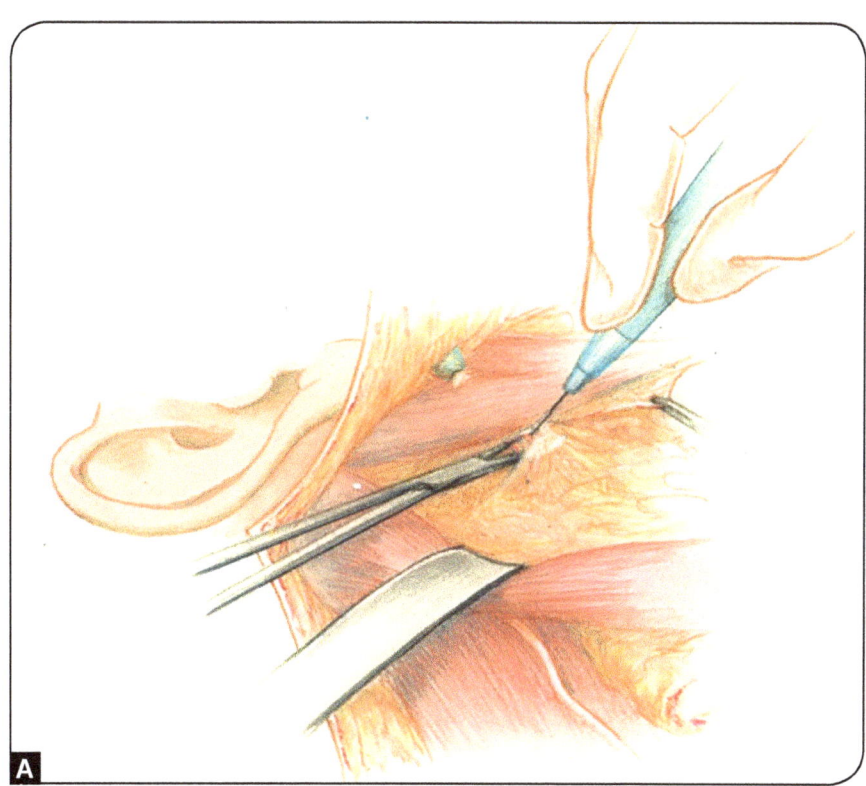

Fig. 2A

- *2B*: This maneuver is repeated as needed to expose the upper end of the IJV, the hypoglossal and the spinal accessory nerves. This part of the dissection often requires ligating or clipping small branches of the occipital artery going in the direction of the SCMM and small tributaries of the IJV; if bleeding occurs while doing this, hurried efforts to control it by clamping in a bloody field jeopardize the hypoglossal nerve.

- *2C*: The dissection is then continued along the posterior border of the strap muscles defining the anterior-inferior limit of the dissection and exposing the superior thyroid vessels and the anterior belly of the omohyoid muscle.

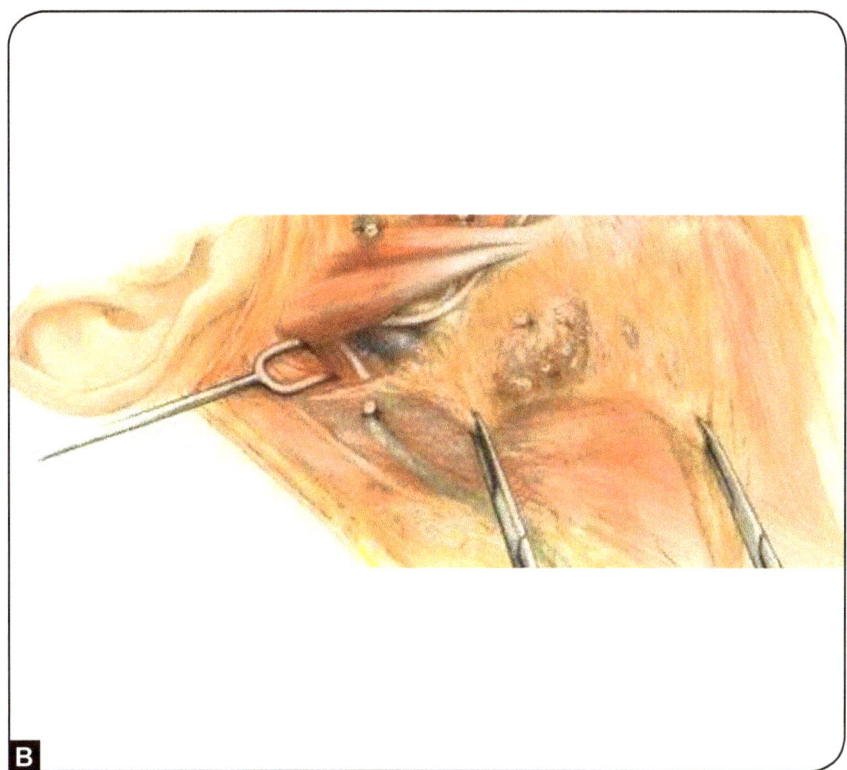

Fig. 2B

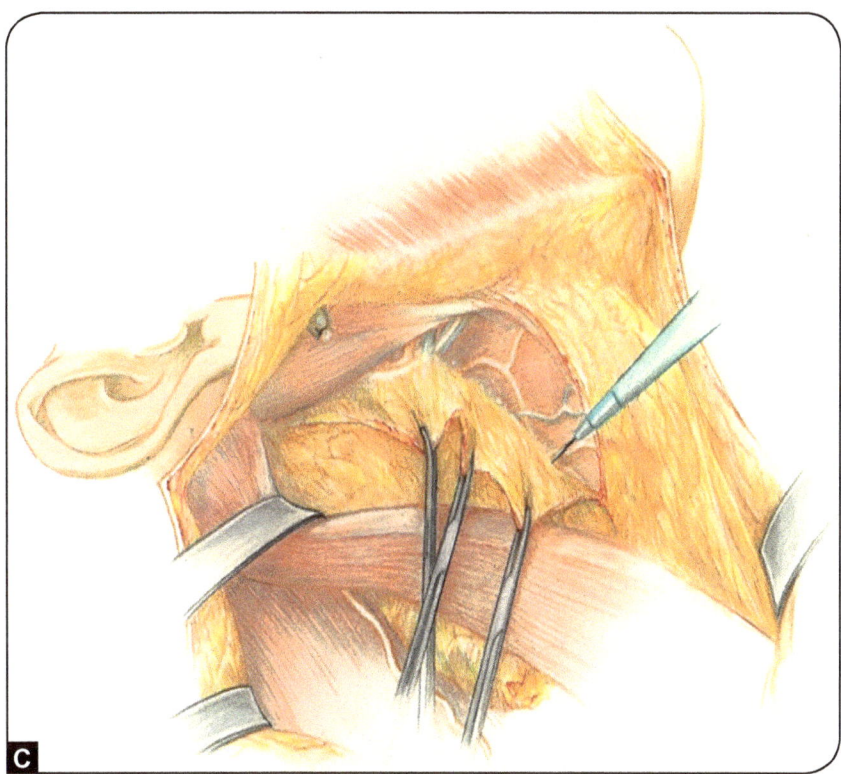

Fig. 2C

- *2D*: The next step consists of dissecting the fascia of the SCMM, beginning where it was previously incised and proceeding in an anterior direction. The dissection of the fascia off of the SCMM continues around the anterior border of the muscle and on to its medial surface. Retracting the muscle laterally, this dissection continues until the spinal accessory nerve is exposed, as it enters the muscle, at about the level of the junction of its upper and middle thirds (arrow).

- *2E*: The fibro-fatty tissue overlying the spinal accessory nerve is then incised using a hemostat to dissect and elevate the tissue over the nerve to protect it. Often, the dissection must be carried around one or more lymph nodes that overlie the nerve. Needless to say that it is paramount to avoid incising these nodes since they can contain metastatic tumors.

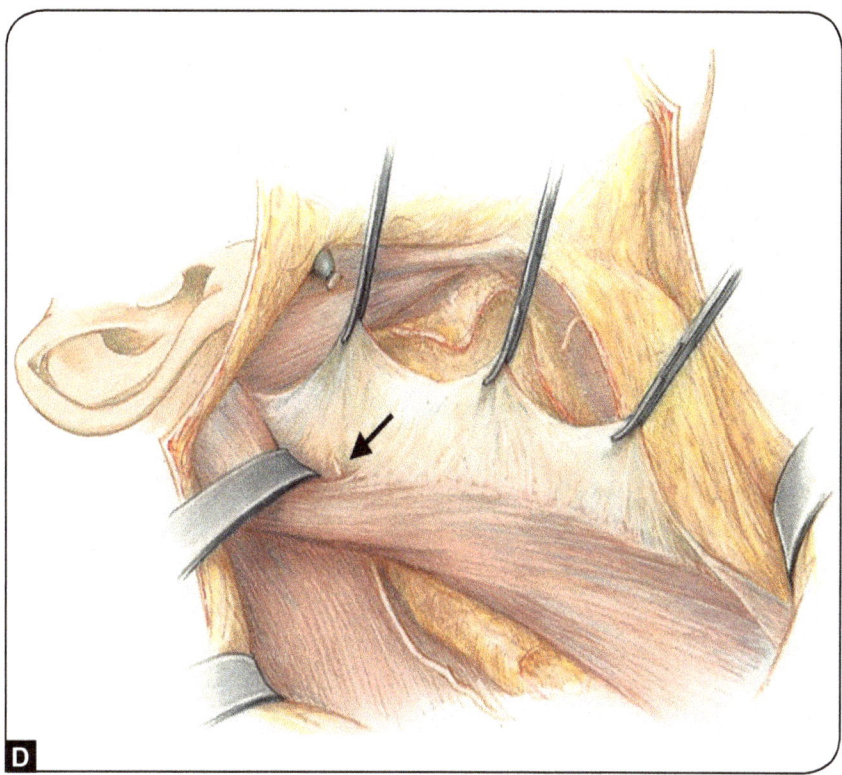

Fig. 2D

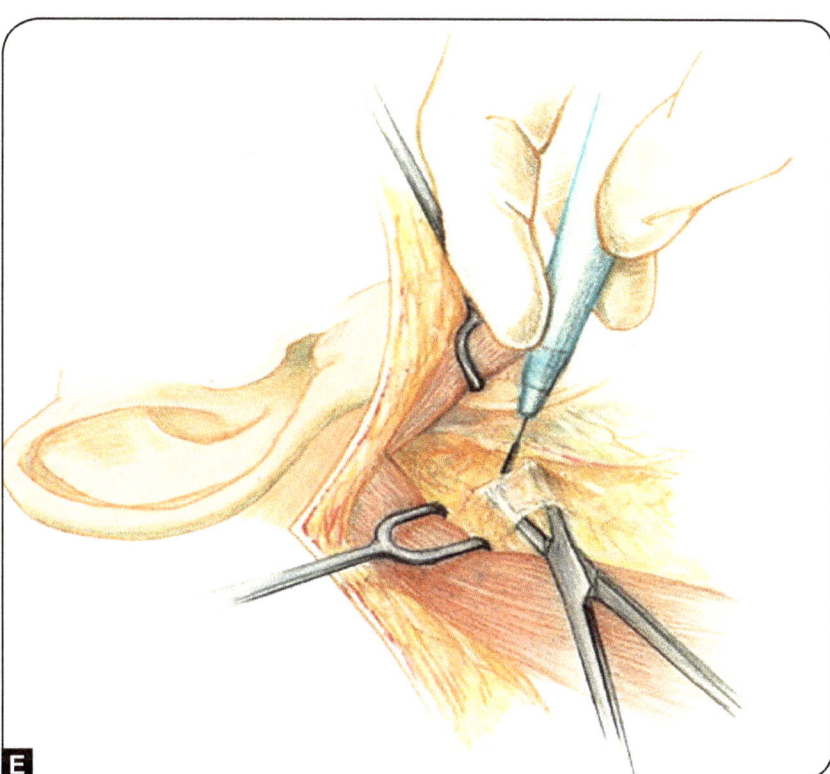

Fig. 2E

▪ *2F*: The nerve is thus exposed between its exit at the jugular foramen and its entrance into the SCMM.

▪ *2G:* The dissection proceeds above and behind the spinal accessory nerve. The fatty tissue of this area is incised along the inferior border of the digastric and then, as far back as possible, in a direction parallel to the posterior border of the SCMM. Then, the fibro-fatty tissue containing lymph nodes is dissected forward, off the splenius capitis and the levator scapulae muscles.

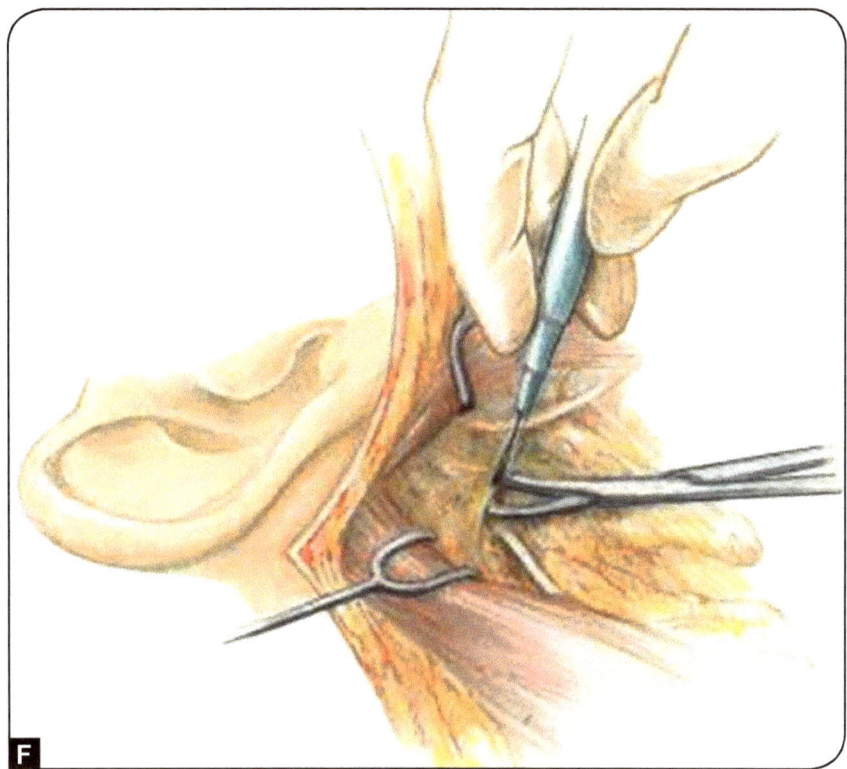

Fig. 2F

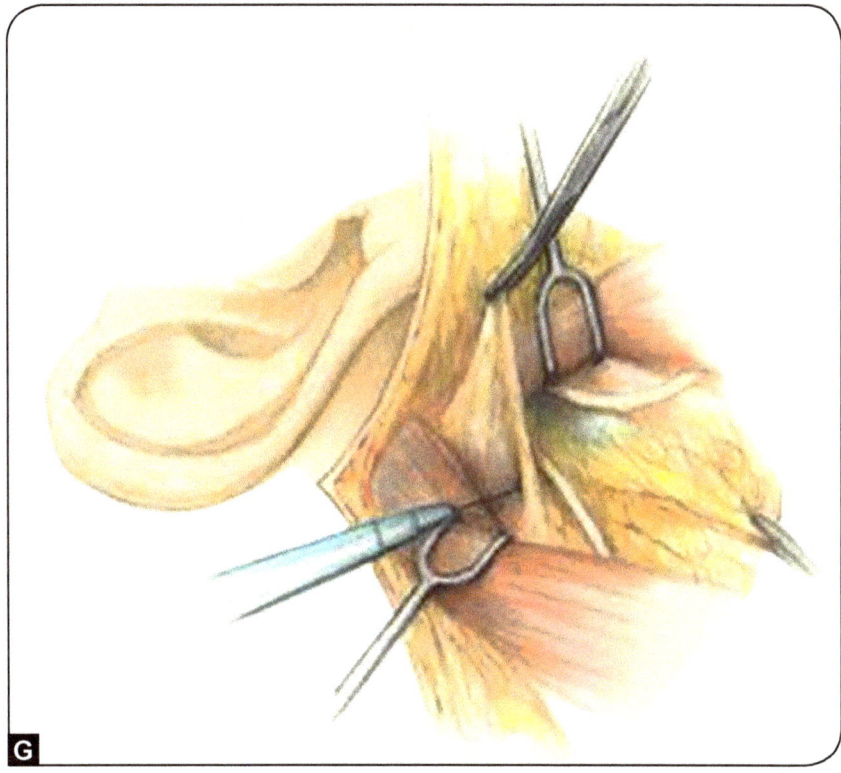

Fig. 2G

- *2H*: The dissected tissue from this area of the neck is brought forward under the spinal accessory nerve.

- *2I*: Below the level of the nerve, the previously freed contents of the posterior triangle are brought forward under the SCMM.

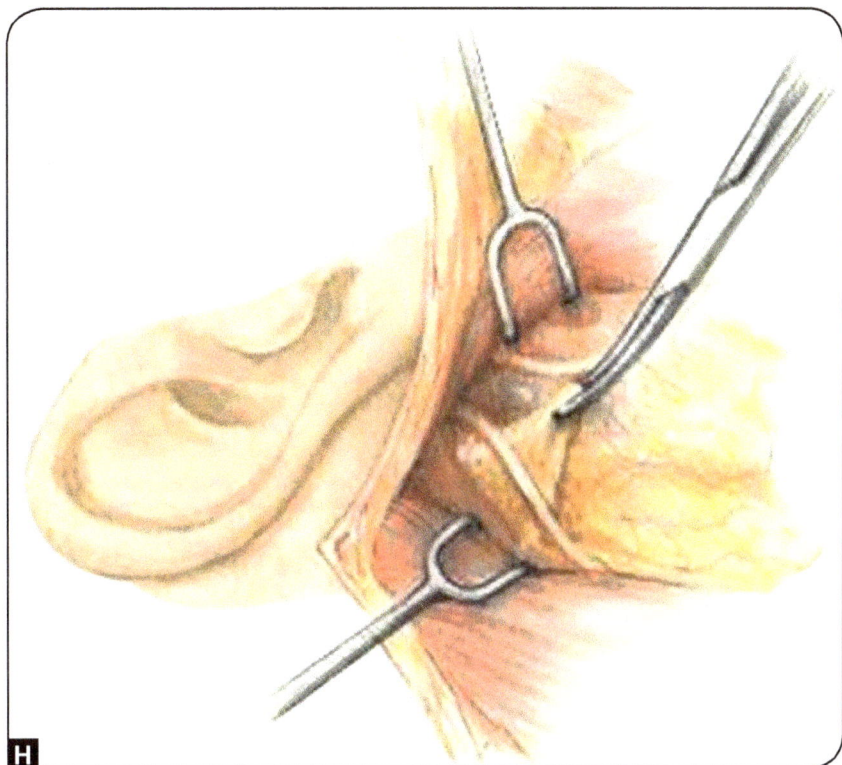

Fig. 2H

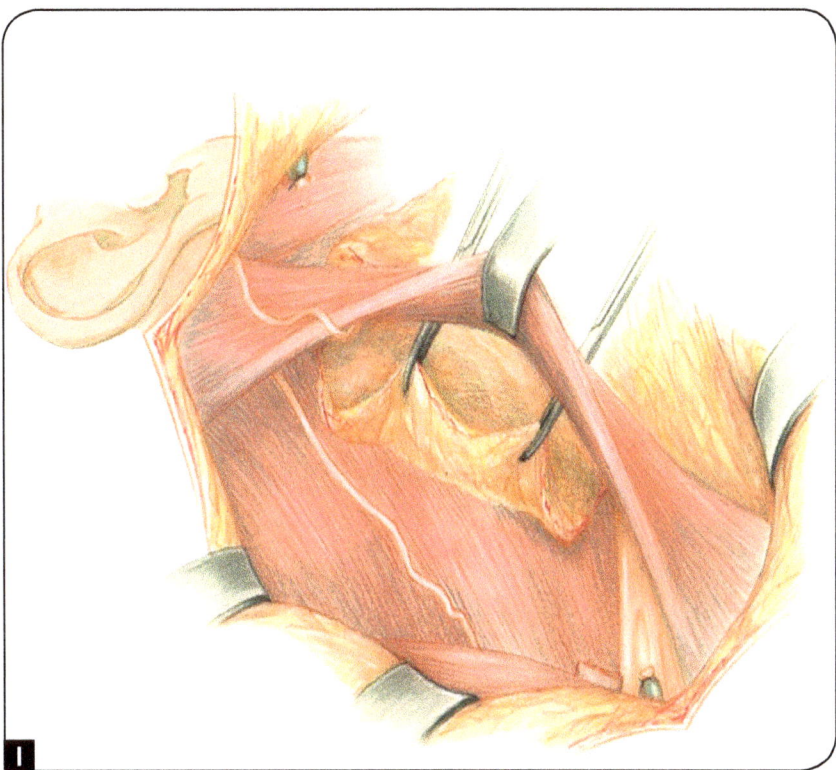

Fig. 2I

- *2J*: The dissection continues in an anterior direction, dividing the inferior cutaneous branches of the cervical plexus. Notice that in this process, the branches of the cervical plexus to the levator scapula muscle should be preserved whenever possible; to do so, the dissection must be carried in a plane lateral or superficial to the fascia of the levator. The specimen is now dissected sharply from the vagus nerve, the carotid artery and the IJV. To avoid injury to the thoracic duct, the dissection in the anterior-inferior area of the neck, lateral to the IJV and the common carotid artery, is carried out carefully, as described in the radical neck dissection (Chapter 3, Section 6A).

- *2K*: The dissection of the specimen from the IJV proceeds superiorly and the anterior belly of the omohyoid muscle is divided usually as it crosses the IJV.

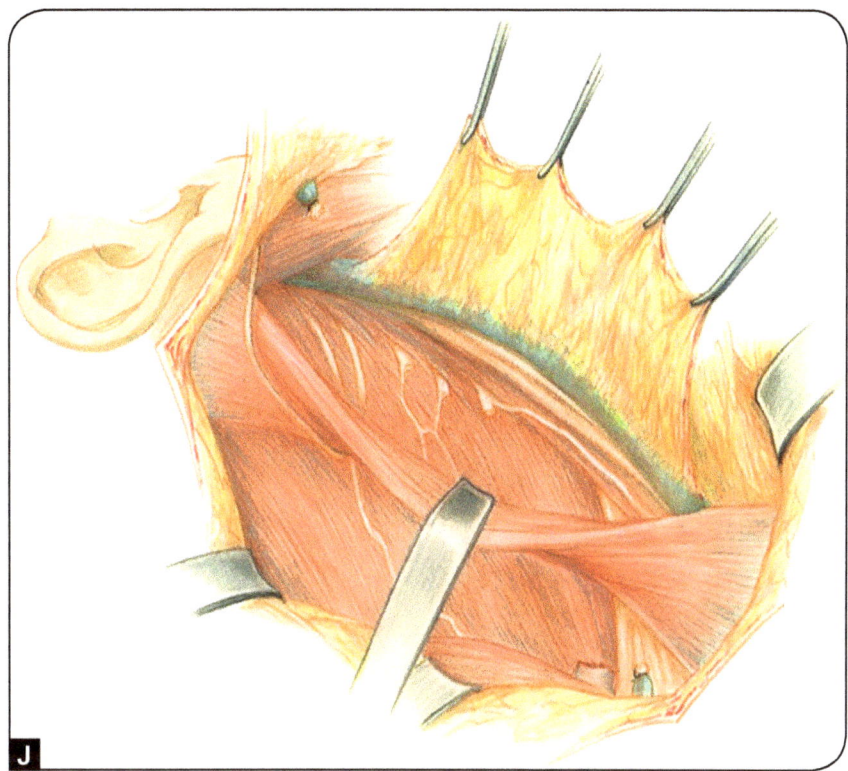

Fig. 2J

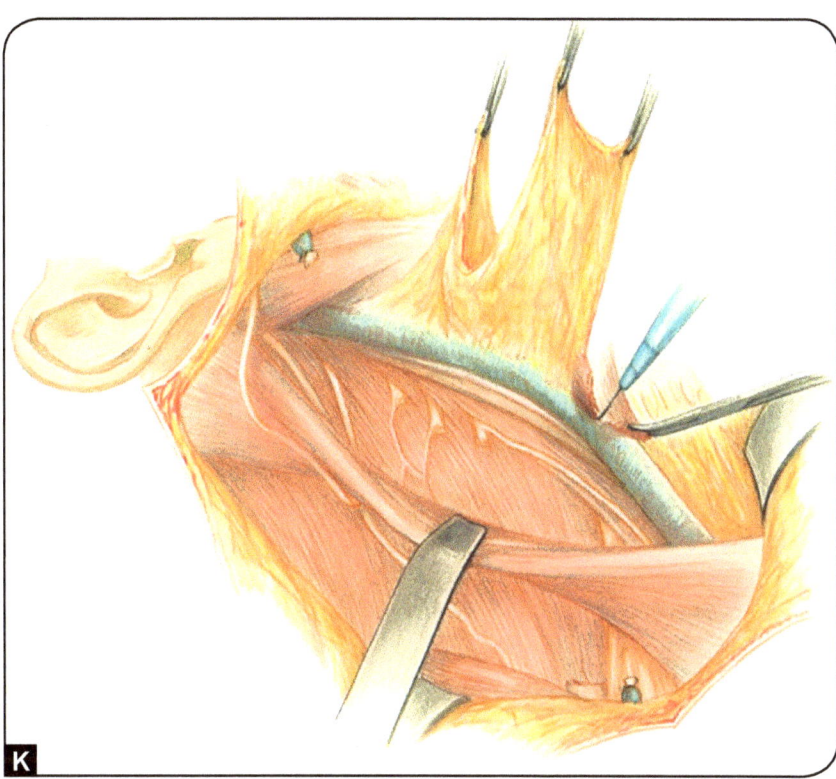

Fig. 2K

- *2L*: At this point of the dissection, the area of the neck between the strap muscles and the IJV is completed preserving, in this case, the superior thyroid vessels.

- *2M*: More often than not, below the level of the hypoglossal nerve, an anterior facial vein or some combination of facial, lingual and thyroid veins must be divided and ligated before the specimen can be removed.

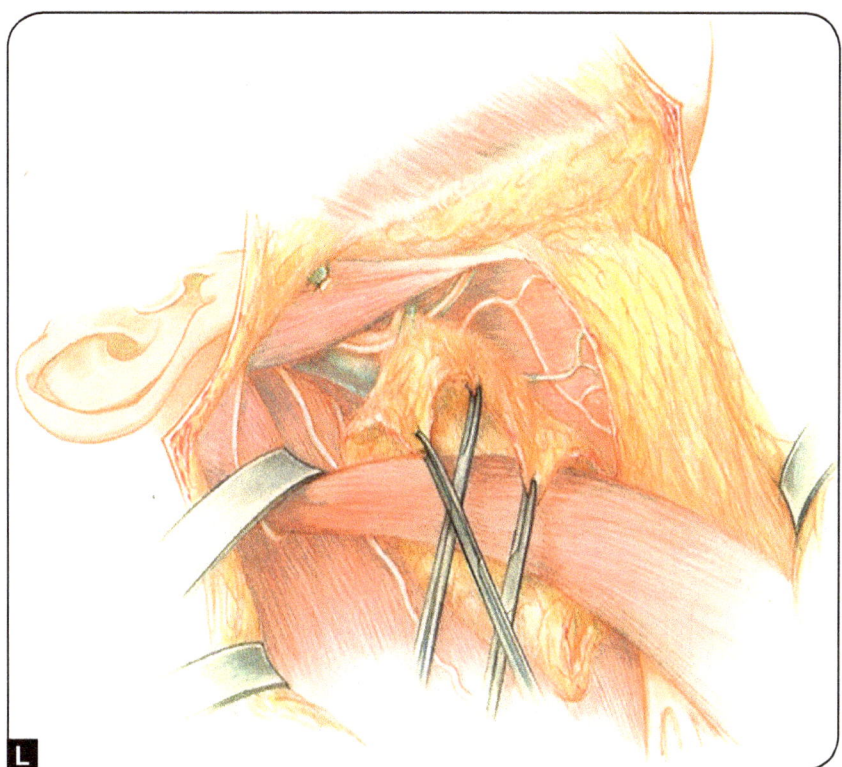

Fig. 2L

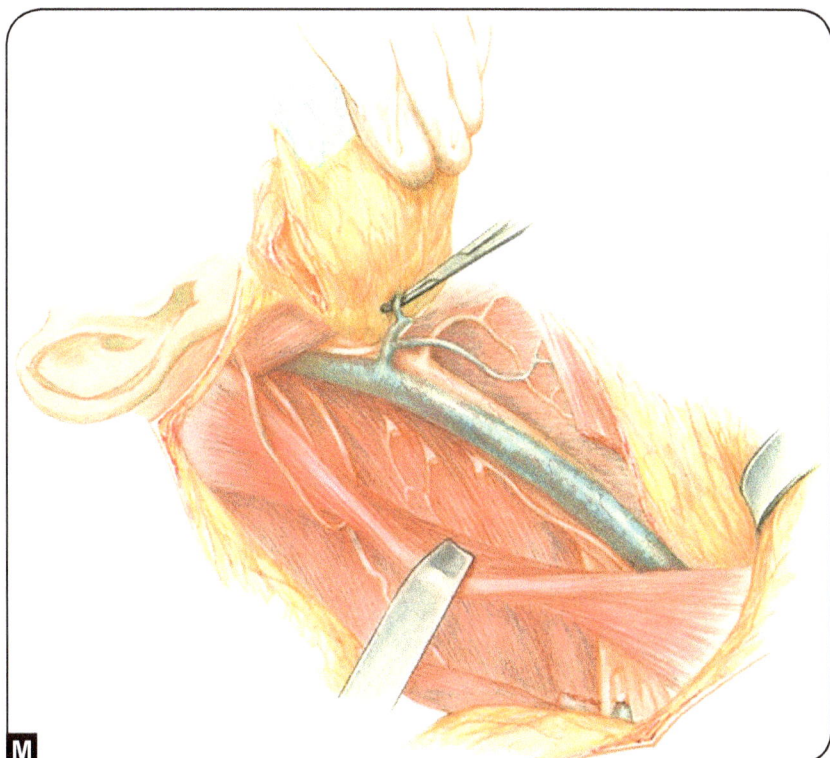

Fig. 2M

- *2N*: The completed dissection extends from the posterior belly of the digastric muscle superiorly to the clavicle inferiorly and from the posterior border of the strap muscles anteriorly to the anterior border of the trapezius muscle.

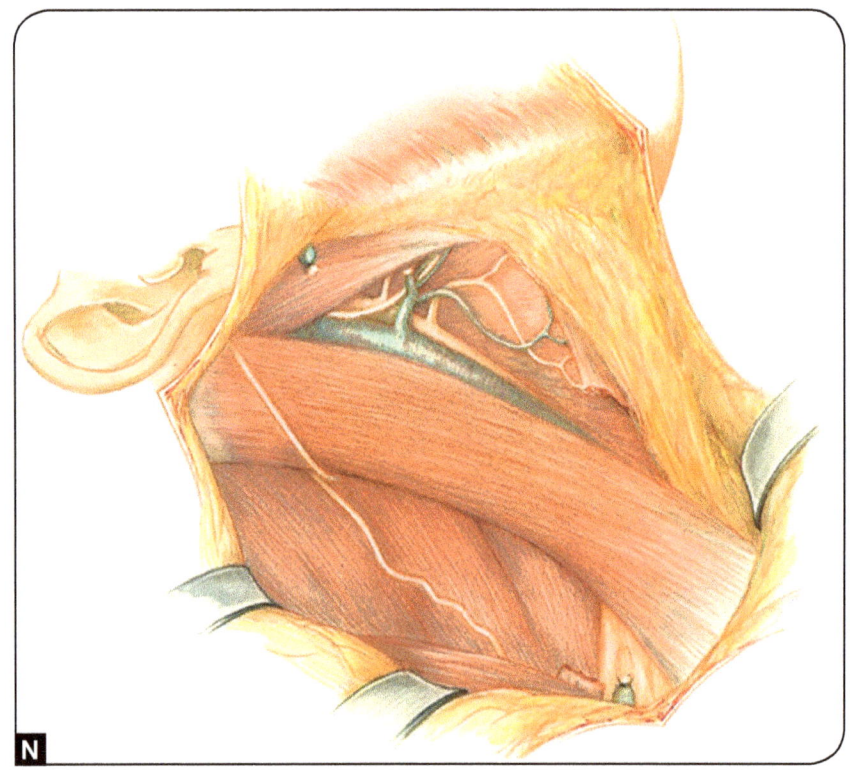

Fig. 2N: Completed MRND preserving the SCMM, IJV, XIN.

REFERENCES

1. Suarez O. El problema de las metastasis linfaticas y alejadas del cancer de laringe e hipofaringe. Rev Otorhinolaringol. 1963;23:83-9.
2. Ferlito A, Rinaldo A. Osvaldo Suarez: often-forgotten father of functional neck dissection (in the non-Spanish-speaking literature). Laryngoscope. 2004;114(7):1177-8.
3. Miodonski J. Treatment of laryngeal cancer. Otolaryngol Pol. 1954;150:503-9.
4. Bocca E, Pignataro O. A conservation technique in radical neck dissection. Ann Otol Rhinol Laryngol. 1967;76(5):975-87.
5. Bocca E, Pignataro O, Sasaki CT. Functional neck dissection. A description of operative technique. Arch Otolaryngol. 1980;106(9):524-7.
6. Lingeman RE, Helmus C, Stephens R, et al. Neck dissection: radical or conservative. Ann Otol Rhinol Laryngol. 1977;86(6): 737-44.
7. Molinari R, Cantu G, Chiesa F, Grandi C. Retrospective comparison of conservative and radical neck dissection in laryngeal cancer. Ann Otol Rhinol Laryngol. 1980;89(6): 578-81.
8. Gavilán C, Gavilán J. Five-year results of functional neck dissection for cancer of the larynx. Arch Otolaryngol Head Neck Surg. 1989;115(10):1193-6.
9. Bocca E, Pignataro O, Oldini C, et al. Functional neck dissection: an evaluation and review of 843 cases. Laryngoscope. 1984;94(7):942-5.

CHAPTER 7

Selective Neck Dissection I–III/IV
(Supraomohyoid Neck Dissection)

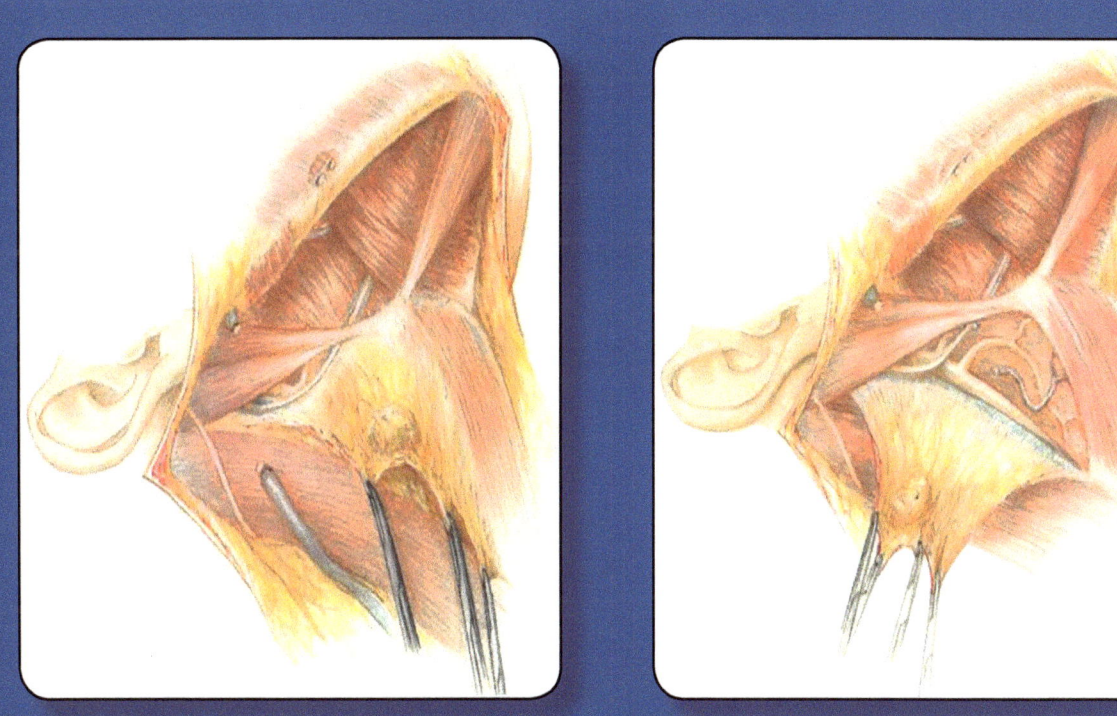

INTRODUCTION

The lymph nodes most frequently involved with metastasis in patients with squamous cell carcinomas of the oral cavity are those in level II and III. In addition, the nodes in level I are frequently involved in patients with carcinoma of the lips, floor of the mouth, anterior oral tongue and buccal mucosa. Furthermore, these tumors frequently metastasize to both sides of the neck, and they can skip levels I and II and metastasize first to level III nodes. In the absence of metastases to the first-echelon nodes, tumors of the oral cavity and oropharynx rarely involve level IV and level V nodes. The nodes in level V are not commonly involved, regardless of the site of the primary tumor and the presence or absence of metastases in the jugular nodes, conceivably because there is no retrograde flow from the jugular nodes into the spinal accessory nodes. In a retrospective study of 1,119 radical neck dissections, Shah[1] found that tumors of the oral cavity metastasized most frequently to the neck nodes in levels I, II and III, whereas carcinomas of the oropharynx, hypopharynx and larynx involved mainly the nodes in levels II, III and IV.

The predictability of lymphatic spread applies to both occult (N0 neck) and clinically evident (N+ neck) lymph node metastases. In an analysis of the distribution of lymph node metastasis in a cohort of 164 patients with oral cancer, who had a single clinically positive node (N1 or N2a), Kowalski and Carvalho[2] found that there were no isolated lymph node metastasis in level IV or V. Furthermore, in patients with tumors of the oral cavity with clinically N1 neck involving level I or II, the affected nodes were histopathologically negative (pN0) in 57.4% of the cases. These findings suggest that a selective neck dissection (SND) of levels I–III could encompass the tumor in the neck in these patients. In other reports, however, the prevalence of metastases in level IV in clinically N+ cases is 17%, suggesting that it is a safer practice to include level IV whenever a SND is done for an N+ neck in patients with cancer of the oral cavity. The prevalence of nodal metastases in level V, on the other hand, is so low in these cases (0.5% in cN0 and 3% in cN+) that dissection of this region of the neck is rarely necessary.[3]

The anatomic and histopathological rational for this type of neck dissection has also translated into outcomes that are comparable to those of more extensive operations. A multi-institutional prospective randomized study comparing the SND I–III to the modified radical neck dissection (MRND) performed by the Brazilian Head and Neck Cancer Study Group[4] showed that in patients with cancer of the oral cavity and clinically N0 neck, the regional control and overall 5-year actuarial survival rates were 87.5% and 67.0% for the supraomohyoid neck dissection (SOHND) group versus 89.5% and 63.0% for the MRND, respectively. The differences were not statistically significant.

INDICATIONS

The SND I–III or IV *(SOHND)* is indicated in the surgical management of the following:[5,6]

- Patients with squamous cell carcinoma of the oral cavity staged T2, T4 and N0, and selected patients with T1N0, i.e. those patients whose tumor is thicker than 4 mm
- Patients with an N1 and selected N2 disease in the neck, particularly when the palpable node is located in level I or level II
- The operation is performed in both sides of the neck in patients with cancers of the anterior tongue and floor of the mouth
- Patients with squamous cell carcinoma of the lip or skin of the midportion of the face who are staged N0, and when these lesions are associated with clinically discrete, single metastases to the submental or submandibular nodes. A bilateral dissection is performed when the lesion is located at or near the midline.

SURGICAL TECHNIQUE

The patient is positioned on the operating table with the neck extended, if necessary, with a roll under the shoulders, the head turned towards the opposite side and stabilized with a foam doughnut.

A unilateral SND I–III is usually performed through a transverse incision located in a crease of the neck. Alternatively, an apron-like incision that extends from the mastoid tip to the mandibular symphysis is used. The lowest point of this incision is usually located at the level of the thyrohyoid membrane. Both of these incisions can be extended into a lip-splitting incision and if a more extensive dissection of the neck is indicated by the surgical findings, a descending limb can be easily added for exposure. Occasionally, it is necessary to excise a scar from a previous lymph node biopsy. In that case, a modification of the Schobinger incision is used. To perform a bilateral dissection, a transverse incision located in a skin crease at an appropriate level is the most commonly used incision. Also, commonly used is an apron-like incision made from mastoid to mastoid overlying the thyrohyoid membrane.

Dissection of the Submandibular and Submental Triangles

This part of the operation is performed as described in Sections 2A–2J of Chapter 3, Radical Neck Dissection.

Superior Lateral Dissection: Level IIA

Steps of superior lateral dissection (level IIa) are as follows:
- *1A*: The dissection of level IIa is crucial, since the majority of metastases occur to the nodes in this level; also, the majority of recurrences after any neck dissection occur in this area of the neck. Therefore, it is important to do this part pristinely avoiding transection of any lymph node.

  The dissection of this area begins by exposing the posterior belly of the digastric muscle. To do this, the inferior most portion of the parotid gland may be dissected and retracted superiorly or transected, if necessary, particularly if in the course of the procedure, the surgeon feels an enlarged or hardened node in the area. It is important then to provide an adequate tissue margin above such a suspicious node.

  The next step is to expose the upper most portion of the internal jugular vein, the spinal accessory nerve and the hypoglossal nerve. To accomplish this safely, the "fascia" overlying the tissues immediately below the inferior border of the muscle is elevated using gentle dissection with a hemostat placed parallel to the muscle. The hemostat is opened and raised slightly allowing the surgeon to incise the elevated tissue without injuring underlying structures.

- *1B*: This maneuver is repeated as many times, as it is needed to expose the desired structures. More often than not, this part of the dissection requires ligating or clipping small branches of the occipital artery going in the direction of the sternocleidomastoid muscle and small tributaries of the internal jugular vein, which can be easily torn causing bleeding and hurried efforts to control it by clamping in a bloody field jeopardize the hypoglossal nerve.

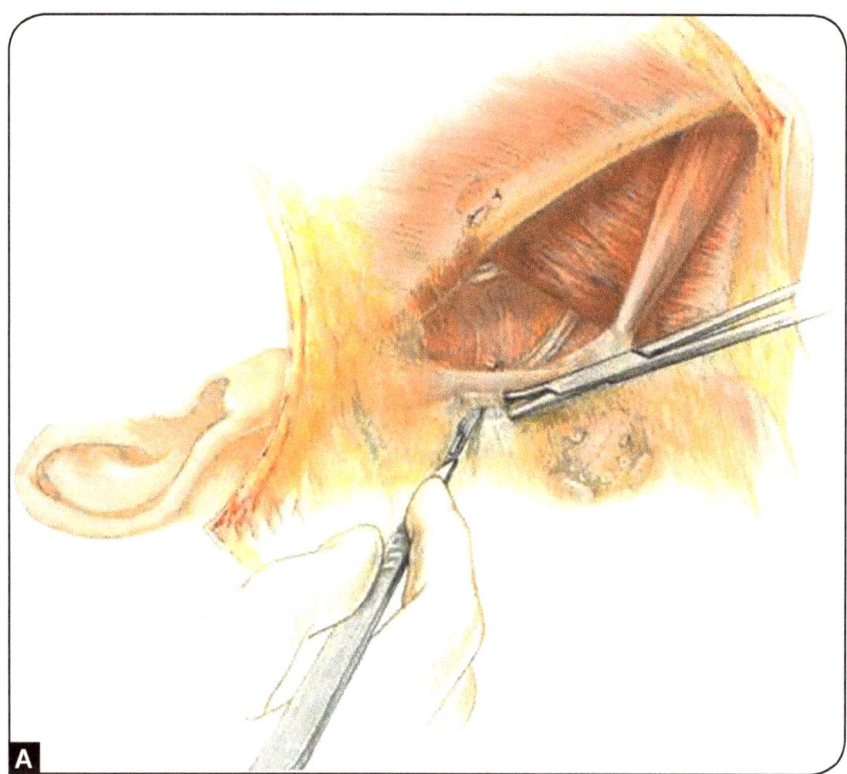

Fig. 1A

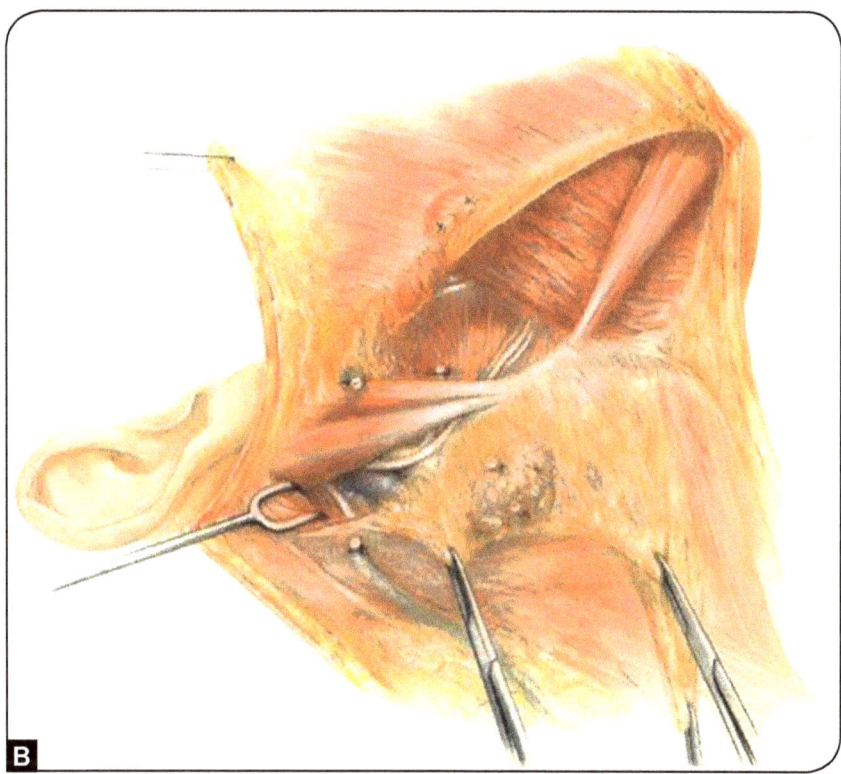

Fig. 1B

- *1C*: Continuing the dissection below the digastric and along the omohyoid muscle, all the fibroadipose tissue in this area is removed, defining the anterior-inferior limit of the dissection.

- *1D*: The dissection is carried posteriorly as far as possible. The superior thyroid vessels are usually preserved. If feasible, the anterior and lateral aspects of the internal jugular vein are exposed, as far down as possible towards the area where the omohyoid crosses it.

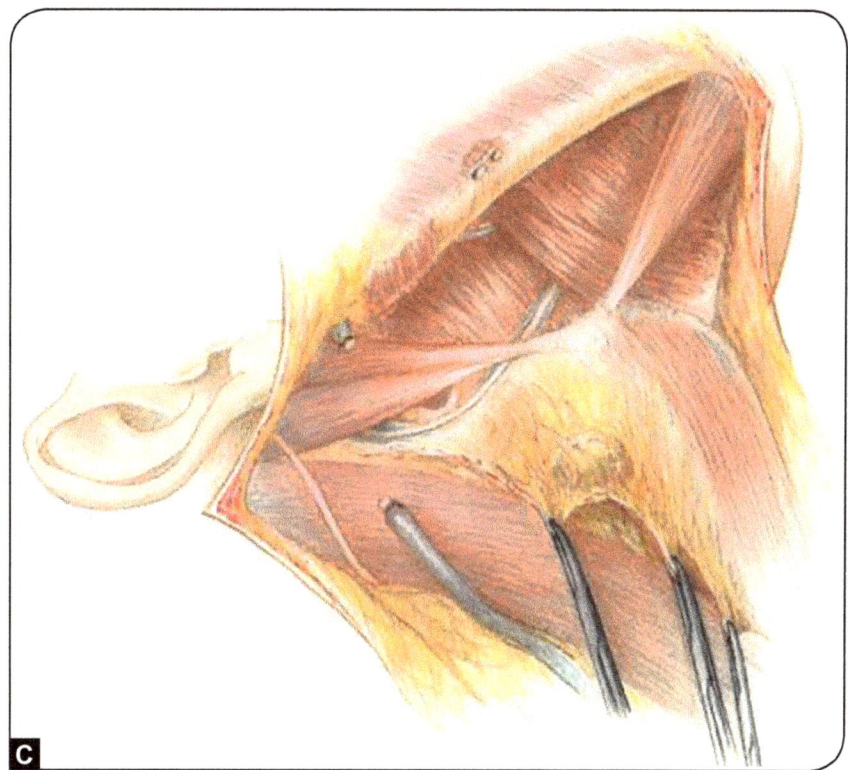

Fig. 1C

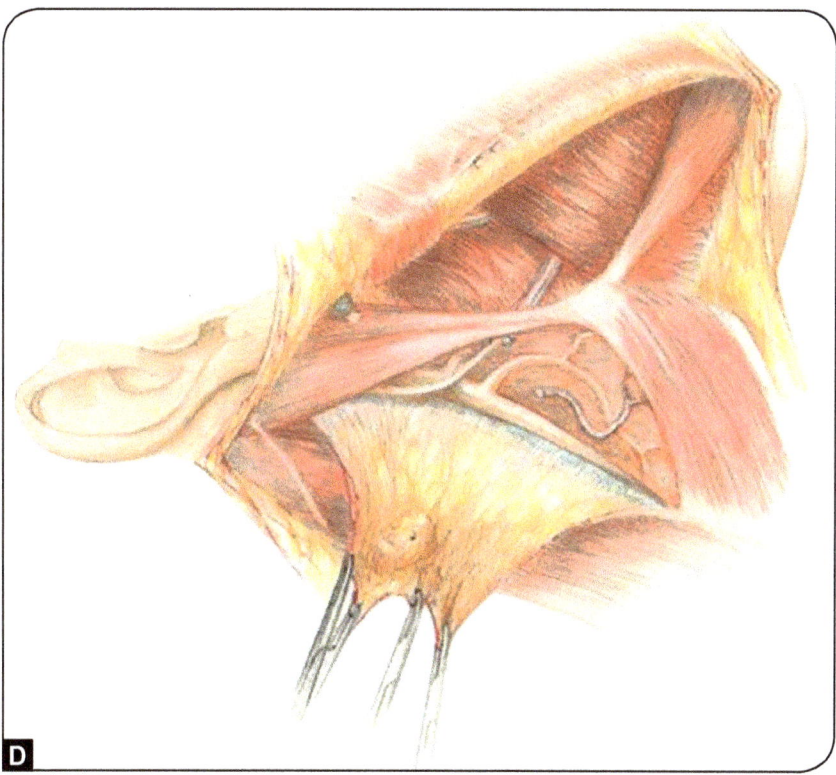

Fig. 1D

- *1E*: The fascia of the sternocleidomastoid muscle is grasped with hemostats along the anterior border of the muscle, down to the level of the omohyoid muscle. In doing so, the external jugular vein is usually divided, unless it is located high enough that it can be preserved without jeopardizing the exposure needed under the sternocleidomastoid muscle. The greater auricular nerve is preserved.

- *1F*: The dissection continues around the anterior border and medial aspect of the sternocleidomastoid muscle until the spinal accessory nerve is exposed superiorly (arrow). Usually, a couple of small vessels entering the muscle obliquely are encountered immediately lateral of inferior to the nerve. Visualizing these nerves warns the surgeon about the proximity of the nerve. Below the nerve, this dissection continues up the level of the posterior border of the muscle.

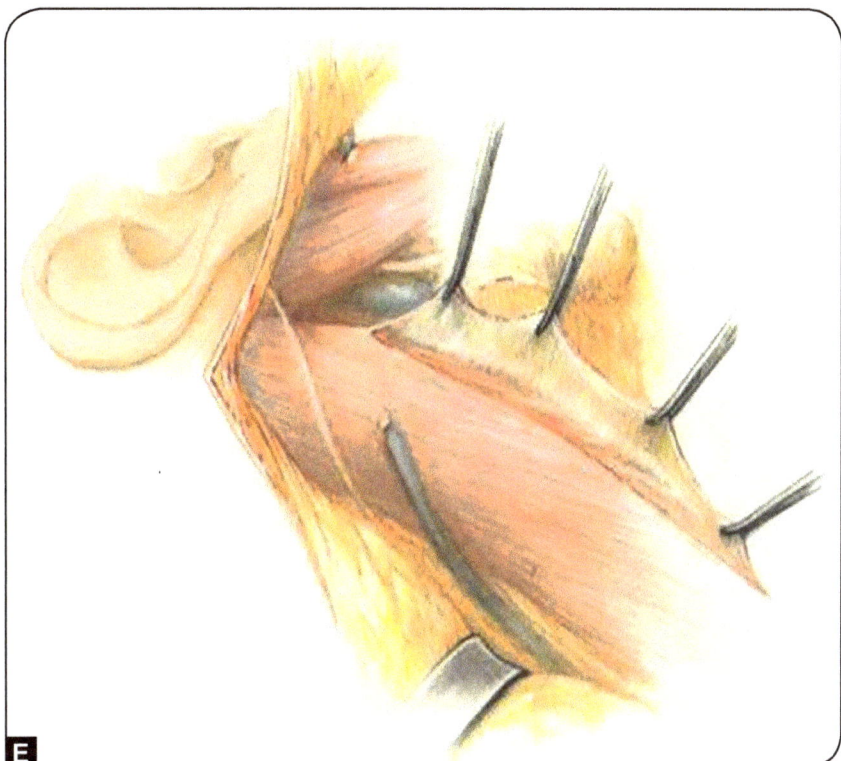

Fig. 1E

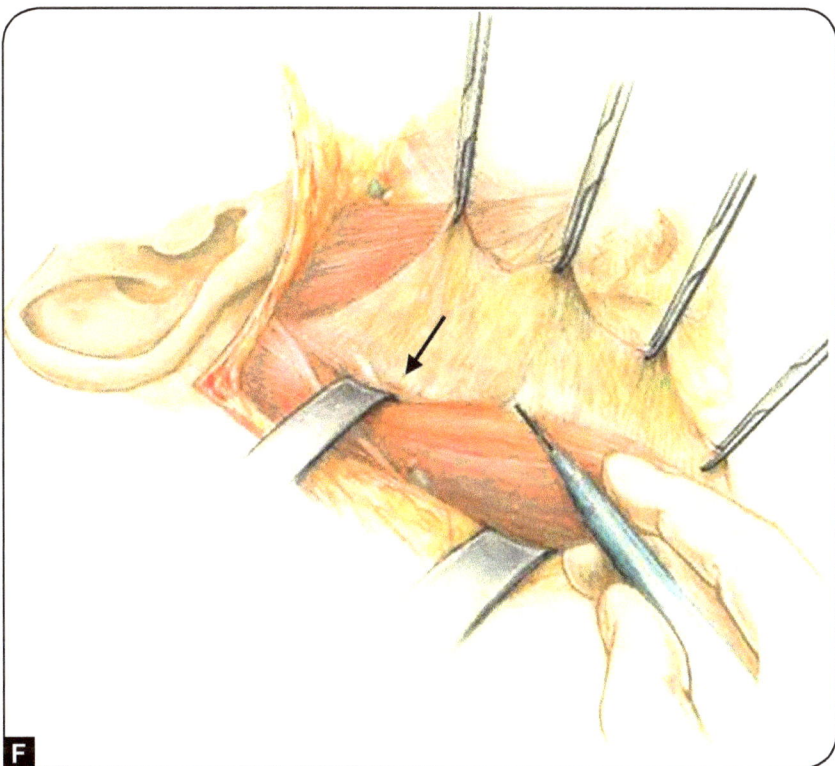

Fig. 1F

- *1G*: Using a hemostat to lift up the tissue lateral to the nerve, the fibro-fatty tissue in the area is incised. The dissection is carried superiorly, up to the level of the digastric; in doing this, care must be taken not to incise through a lymph node. Visualization of the lymph nodes is facilitated by keeping the field bloodless using the monopolar and bipolar cautery.

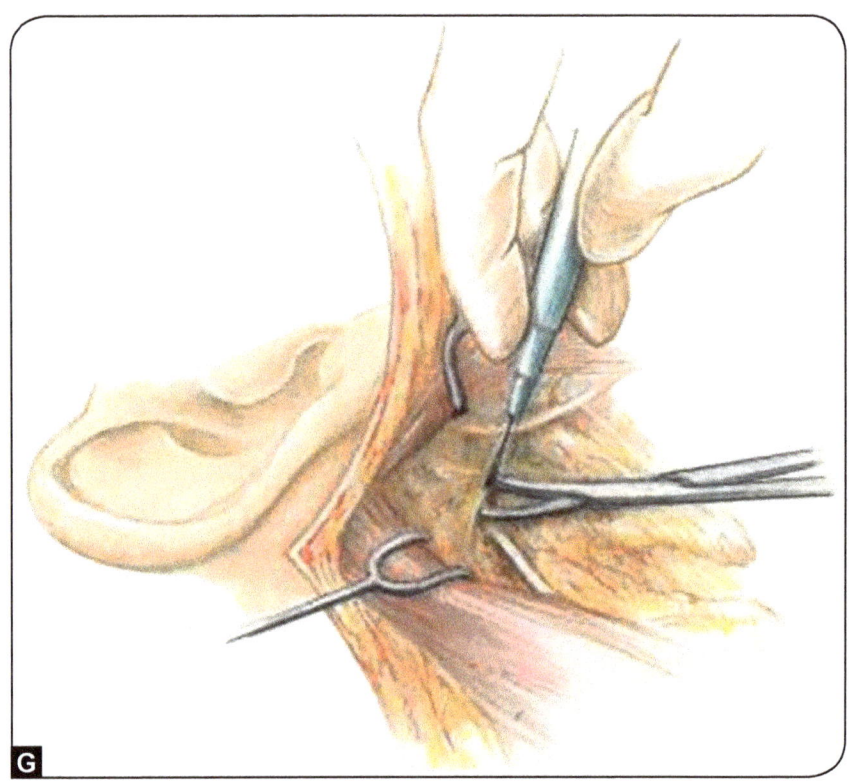

Fig. 1G

Dissection of Level IIb

Steps of dissection of level IIb are as follows:
- *2A*: Above the level of the spinal accessory nerve, the sternocleidomastoid muscle is retracted using a Green or a Richardson retractor. The fibro-fatty tissue above and behind the nerve is incised superiorly, below the inferior border of the digastric and, posteriorly, as far back under the sternocleidomastoid muscle as feasible. Once the splenius capitis muscle is reached, the dissection is carried forward over the levator scapulae muscle. In doing this part of the dissection, the surgeon must keep in mind that the levator is not at the same level and in immediate continuity with the splenius. The levator muscle is slightly anterior to the splenius and there is a small hiatus between the two muscles. Thus, when this hiatus is reached, carrying the dissection forward at the level of the splenius muscle may lead the beginning surgeon to a plane behind the levator scapula. That is why, the author fondly calls this area the "valley of the lost resident".
- *2B*: The fine fascia adjacent to the spinal accessory nerve is incised, with a knife, along both sides of the entire length of the exposed nerve; then the fibroadipose tissue containing lymph nodes from this area is brought forward underneath the spinal accessory nerve.

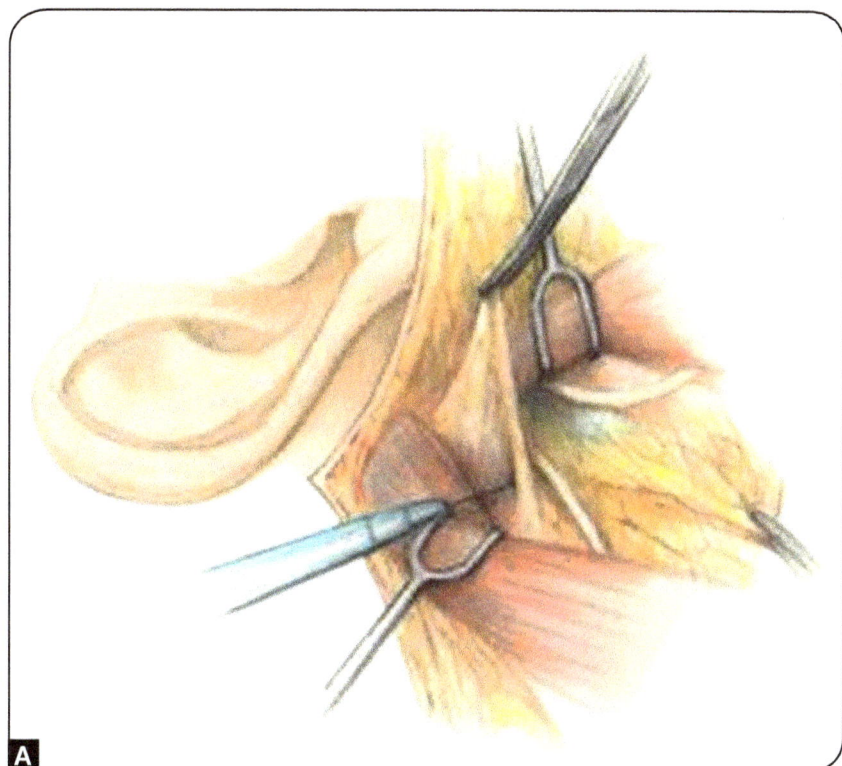

Fig. 2A

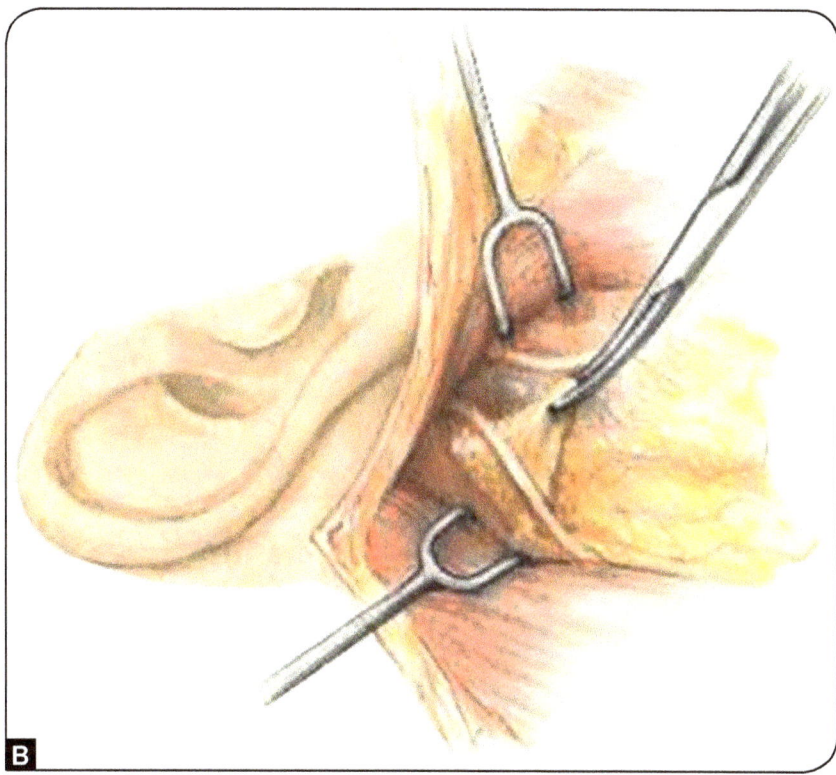

Fig. 2B

Dissection of Level III

Steps of dissection of level III are as follows:

- *3A*: Below the spinal accessory nerve, the posterior limit of the dissection is marked by the cutaneous branches of the cervical plexus, as they reach the posterior border of the sternocleidomastoid muscle, where they are identified and preserved. A block of adipose tissue containing lymph nodes is thus formed, which is reflected anteriorly and dissected off the cervical plexus roots or nerves, the levator scapulae muscle and the upper portion of the medial and scalene muscles.

- *3B*: The dissection is then carried along the carotid compartment, from posterior to anterior, identifying and preserving the vagus nerve and dissecting the specimen sharply from the internal jugular vein. The inferior limit of the dissection is the omohyoid muscle as it crosses forward, lateral to the internal jugular vein. However, if a node is found in this area that appears to be involved by tumor, the omohyoid is retracted downwards or divided, and the lymph nodes and adipose tissue anterior to the scalene muscles and the brachial plexus (lymph node group IV) are included in the specimen.

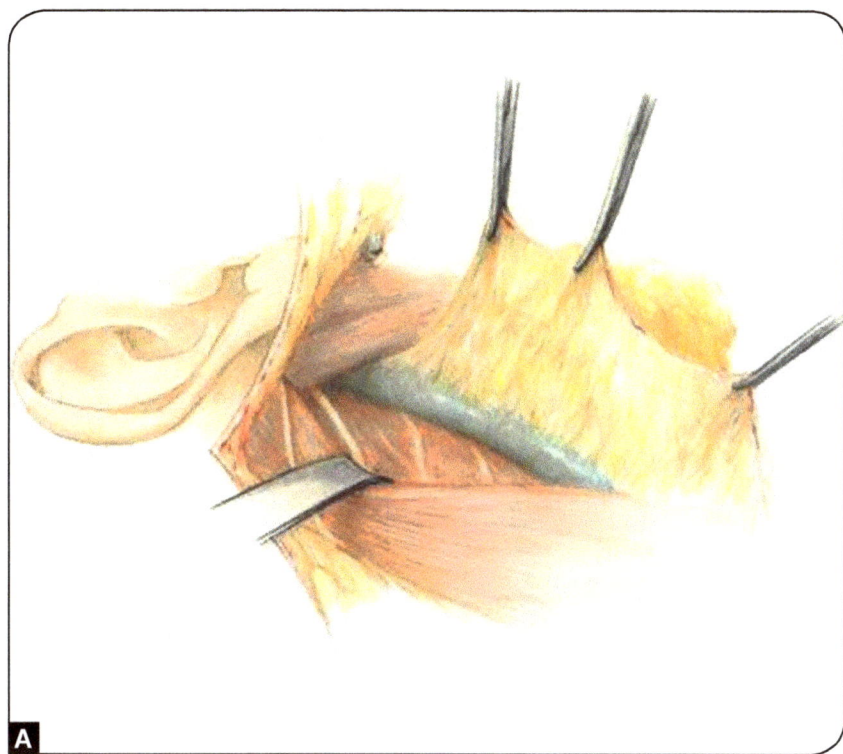

Fig. 3A

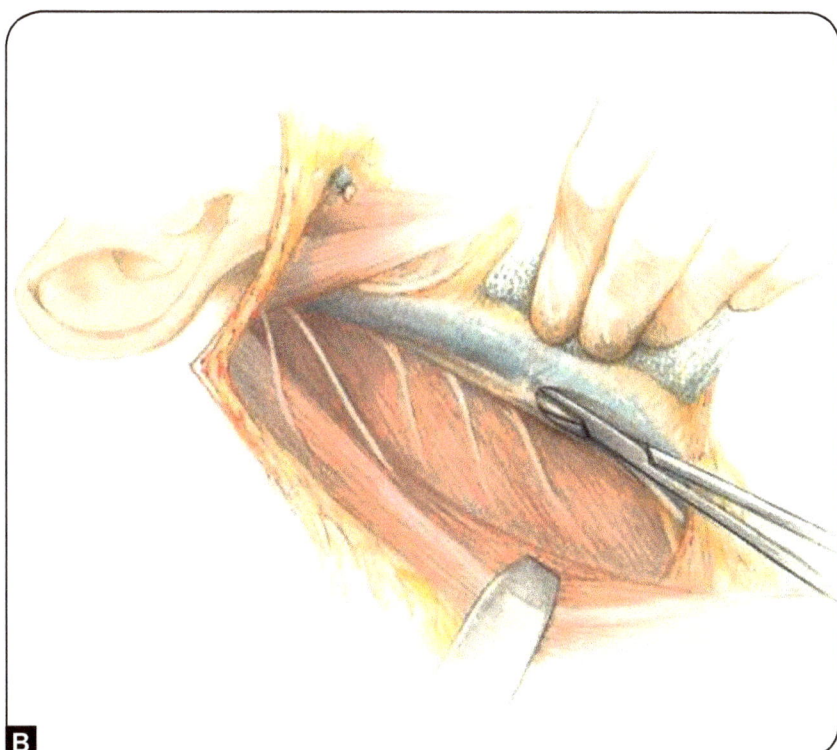

Fig. 3B: The fascia that envelops the vascular compartment has been incised deliberately and a clamp is used to show the position of the vagus nerve relative to the IJV.

- *3C*: More often than not, the common facial vein has to be divided as is shown in Figure 3C and the surgical specimen is dissected from the internal jugular vein. In the vast majority of cases, it is not necessary or advisable to dissect the vein circumferentially or to dissect deeply, anterior and medial to the vein where the common carotid artery is located.

- *3D*: The specimen has been removed and all the structures preserved are clearly shown. When the dissection is completed, only a small amount of lymph node-bearing tissue remains in the posterior-inferior aspect of the neck. In cases that require a bilateral neck dissection, the specimen is dissected off of the strap muscles up to the midline and onto the other side of the neck.

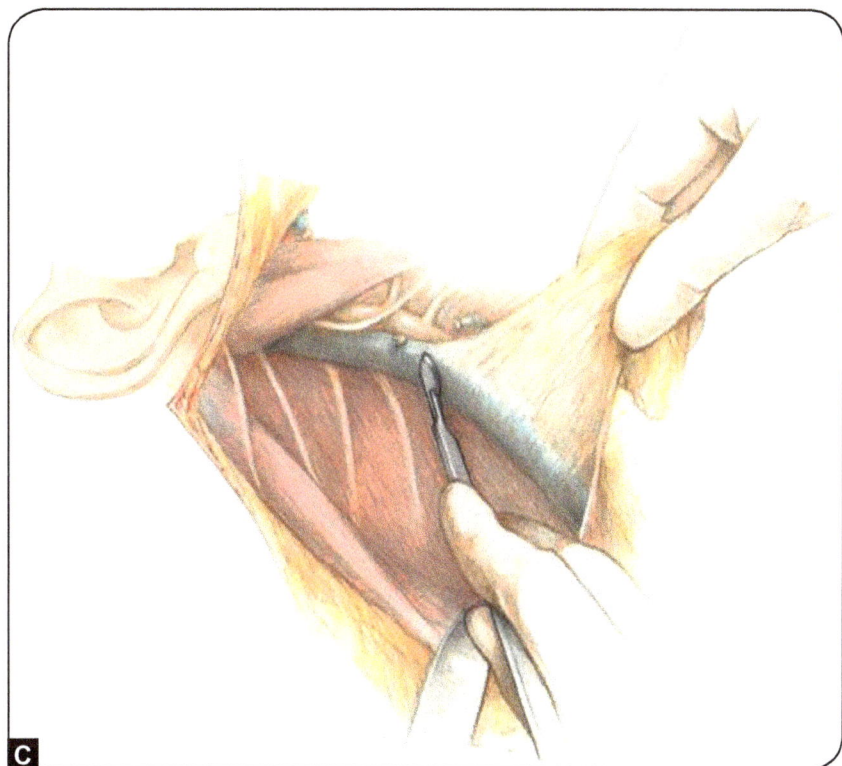

Fig. 3C

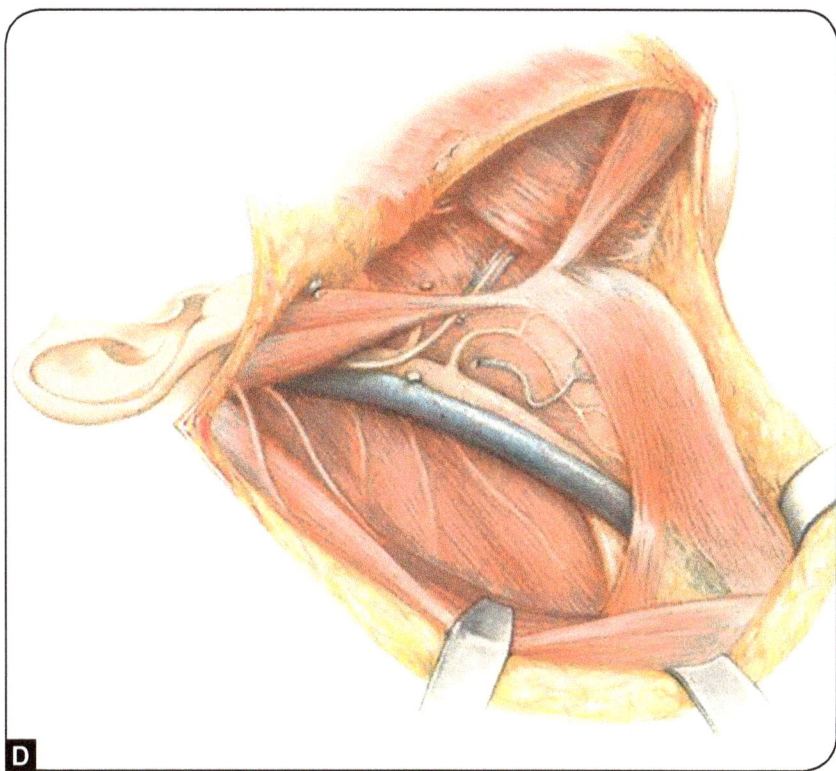

Fig. 3D: Completed SND I-III.

REFERENCES

1. Shah JP. Patterns of cervical lymph node metastasis from squamous carcinomas of the upper aerodigestive tract. Am J Surg. 1990;160(4):405-9.
2. Kowalski LP, Carvalho AL. Feasibility of supraomohyoid neck dissection in N1 and N2a oral cancer patients. Head Neck. 2002;24(10):921-4.
3. Shah JP, Candela FC, Poddar AK. The patterns of cervical lymph node metastases from squamous cell carcinoma of the oral cavity. Cancer. 1990;66(1):109-13.
4. Results of a prospective trial on elective modified radical classical versus supraomohyoid neck dissection in the management of oral squamous carcinoma. Brazilian Head and Neck Cancer Study Group. Am J Surg. 1998;176(5):422-7.
5. Andersen PE, Warren F, Spiro J, et al. Results of selective neck dissection in management of the node-positive neck. Arch Otolaryngol Head Neck Surg. 2002;128(10):1180-4.
6. Patel RS, Clark JR, Gao K, et al. Effectiveness of selective neck dissection in the treatment of the clinically positive neck. Head Neck. 2008;30(9):1231-6.

CHAPTER 8

Selective Neck Dissection II–IV
(Lateral Neck Dissection)

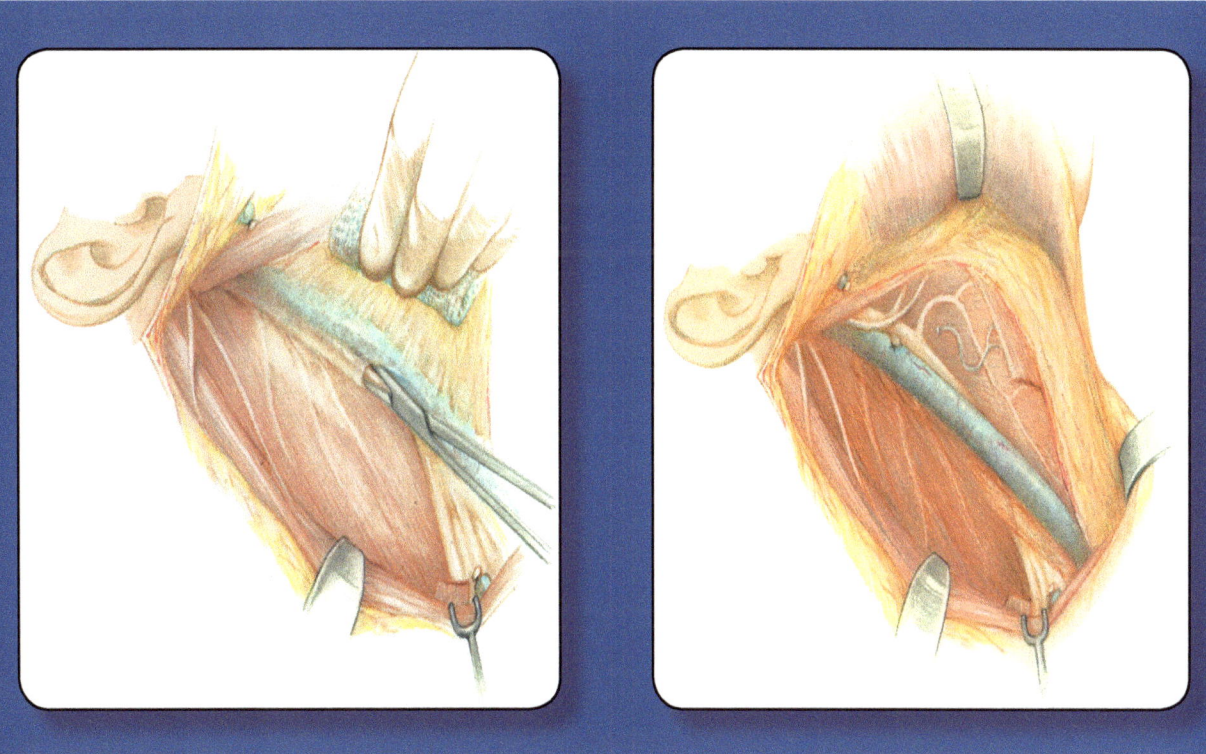

INTRODUCTION

The lymphatics of the supraglottic region cover the entire laryngeal surface of the epiglottis, the false cords and the aryepiglottic folds in a continuous network, which communicate with the lymphatic network of the base of the tongue and the hypopharynx. Because of these features, tumors in the supraglottic larynx have the potential to metastasize to lymph nodes of both sides of the neck. The lymphatic drainage from the supraglottic larynx occurs primarily to the ipsilateral level II and III nodes and to a lesser extent to the contralateral lymph nodes.[1]

A prospective study of the prevalence and distribution of histological lymph node metastases in 100 consecutive neck dissections has shown that metastases in N0 and N1 cases were confined to levels II, III, IV and VI. Metastases to levels I and V were infrequent, even in N+ cases, and occurred only in cases with N2c and N3 disease. These results support the use of a dissection of node levels II–IV for N0 and selected N+ cases with laryngeal and hypopharyngeal cancer.[2]

The regional control and survival rates observed in several retrospective studies suggested that a selective neck dissection (SND) of levels II–IV was as effective as more extensive neck dissections.[3-5] In addition, the inclusion of level V in SNDs for patients with cancer of the larynx has been questioned by a careful analysis of the literature (Rinaldo, 2004 77/id). Furthermore, a multi-institutional prospective randomized study comparing the SND of levels II–IV to the modified radical neck dissection, performed by the Brazilian Head and Neck Cancer Study Group, showed that the 5-year overall survival and neck recurrence rates and complications were similar in both groups.[6]

Finally, the outcomes observed in several clinical and histopathological studies suggest that this type of SND is an appropriate operation in some patients with clinically obvious cervical lymph node metastasis.[7,8]

INDICATIONS

The SND II–IV is indicated in the following situations:
- Patients with cancers of the larynx, oropharynx and hypopharynx staged T2, T4, N0 and N1, who are initially treated with surgery (conventional or transoral surgery), particularly when the possibility that the patient may be treated with surgery alone is considered. Because the lymphatic drainage of these regions is such that metastases are frequently bilateral, the operation is often done on both sides of the neck.
- Patients with carcinomas of the larynx or pharynx undergoing a "planned" neck dissection for residual tumor in the neck, at least 12 weeks after treatment with radiation, with or without chemotherapy. This type of neck dissection is well-suited and effective in patients who have, initially, N1 disease confined to level II and whose residual disease is also confined to level II.[9-11]
- Patients undergoing "salvage" laryngectomy for recurrent cancer after previous treatment with radiation with or without chemotherapy.[11]

SURGICAL TECHNIQUE

The incisions commonly used for this type of neck dissection are the unilateral and bilateral hockey-stick incisions and the mid-transverse incision as described in detail in Chapter 2. Subplatysmal flaps are elevated. However, once the inferior border of the submandibular gland has been identified, no further anterior-superior elevation of the flap is required. The inferior flap should be elevated up to the level of the clavicle. The greater auricular nerve and external jugular vein are usually preserved.

- *1A*: The dissection begins immediately below and posterior to the cervical branch of the facial nerve. If this is not visualized, the dissection begins immediately below the submandibular gland. It is preferable to leave the fascia covering the gland intact. Otherwise, with time, the gland will become ptotic. The tissues are incised in several layers until the posterior belly of the digastric muscle is exposed. As in other neck dissections, depending upon the location and the extent of the tumor in the neck, the tail of the parotid gland may be dissected and retracted superiorly or transected, if necessary, to provide an adequate tissue margin. Likewise, it may be necessary to include the posterior belly of the digastric in the dissected specimen.

- *1B*: The posterior belly of the digastric is slightly retracted upwards with an Army-Navy or a similar retractor. Then, with careful dissection, the uppermost portion of the internal jugular vein, the spinal accessory nerve and the hypoglossal nerve are exposed. A useful technique to accomplish this safely consists of applying gentle inferior traction to the "specimen" and using a fine tip hemostat, such as a mosquito clamp, a thin layer of tissue is pierced; then, changing the angle of the clamp, as needed, the tip of the clamp is gently driven forward, under a thin layer of fascia or tissue. Opening the clamp a few millimeters, and elevating with it a "see-through" layer of tissue allows the surgeon to cut the tissues without injuring the underlying structures. This maneuver is repeated as needed to expose the upper end of the internal jugular vein (IJV), the hypoglossal and the spinal accessory nerves.
  This part of the dissection often requires ligating or clipping small branches of the occipital artery going in the direction of the sternocleidomastoid muscle (SCMM) and small tributaries of the IJV; if bleeding occurs while doing this, it is important for the surgeon not to rush to secure the bleeding vessel with a clamp as the hypoglossal nerve may be injured in the process.

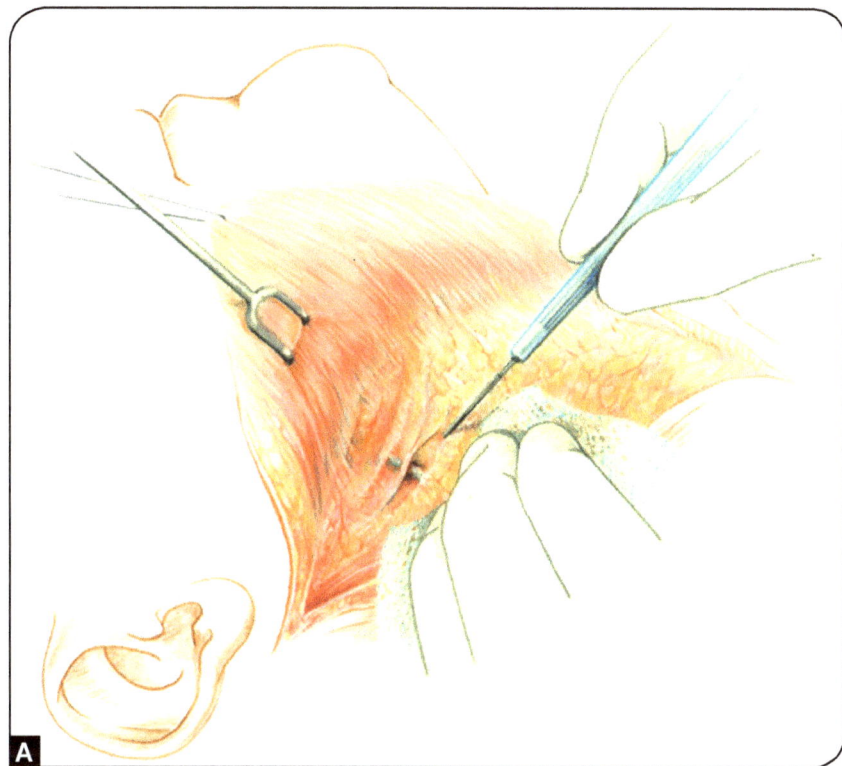

Fig. 1A

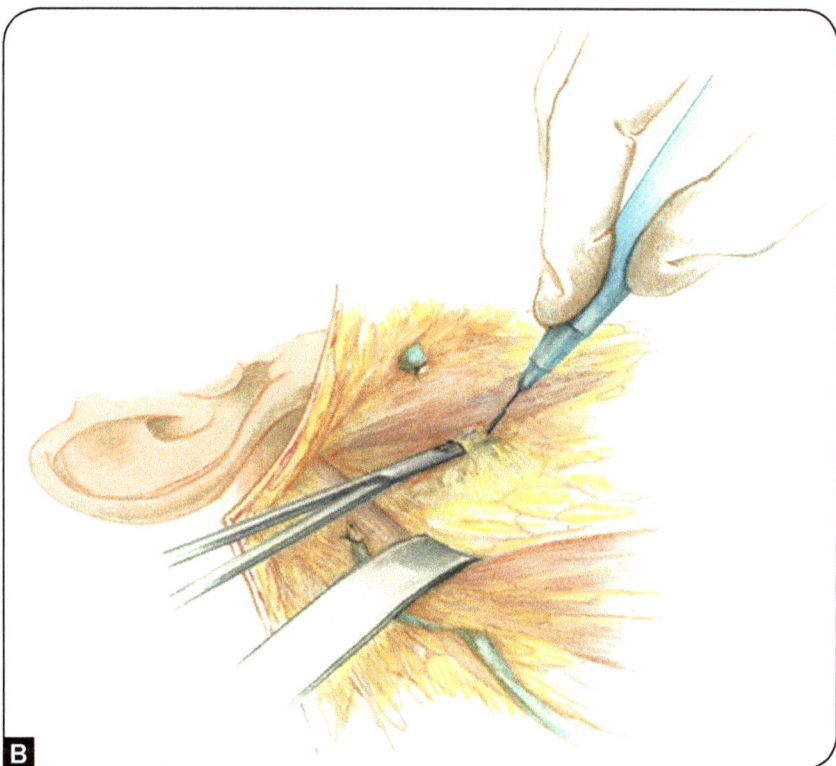

Fig. 1B

- *1C*: The dissection is then continued along the posterior border of the strap muscles defining the anterior-inferior limit of the dissection and exposing the superior thyroid vessels and the anterior belly of the omohyoid muscle.

- *1D*: The external jugular vein is divided. However, if it is located posteriorly enough, it may be preserved. The fascia of the SCMM is grasped with hemostats, along the anterior border of the muscle.
The dissection proceeds circumferentially, around the anterior border of the SCMM, from the clavicle up to the level of the posterior belly of the digastric muscle. Near the middle of the body of the muscle and sometimes closer to its posterior border, at about the level of the junction of the upper and middle thirds of the muscle, the spinal accessory nerve is exposed. As this area is approached, the presence of one or two vessels that enter the SCMM obliquely should alert the surgeon as to the proximity of the spinal accessory nerve.

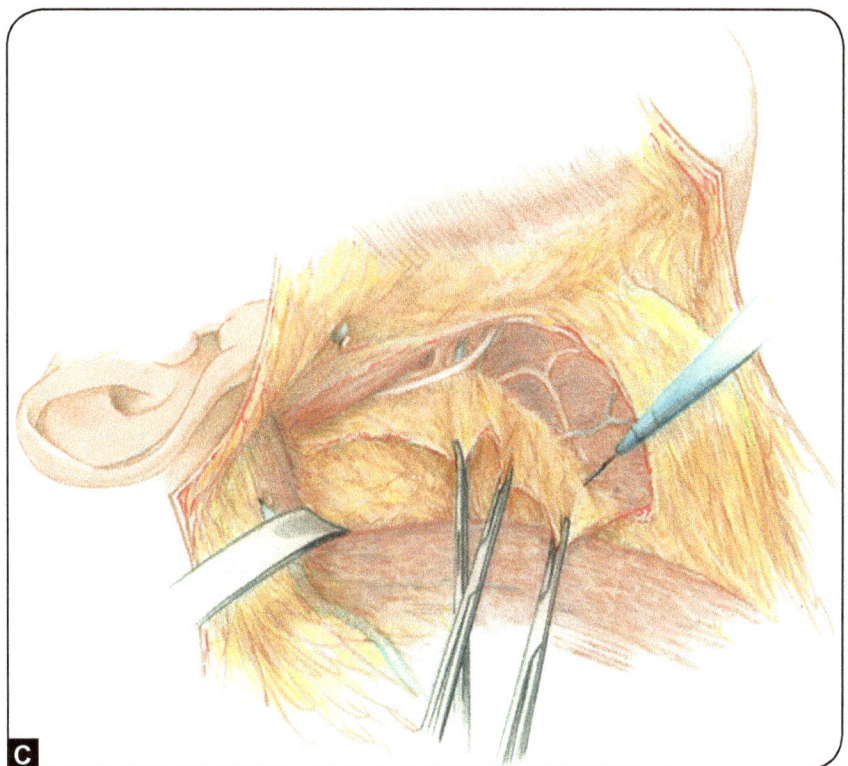

Fig. 1C

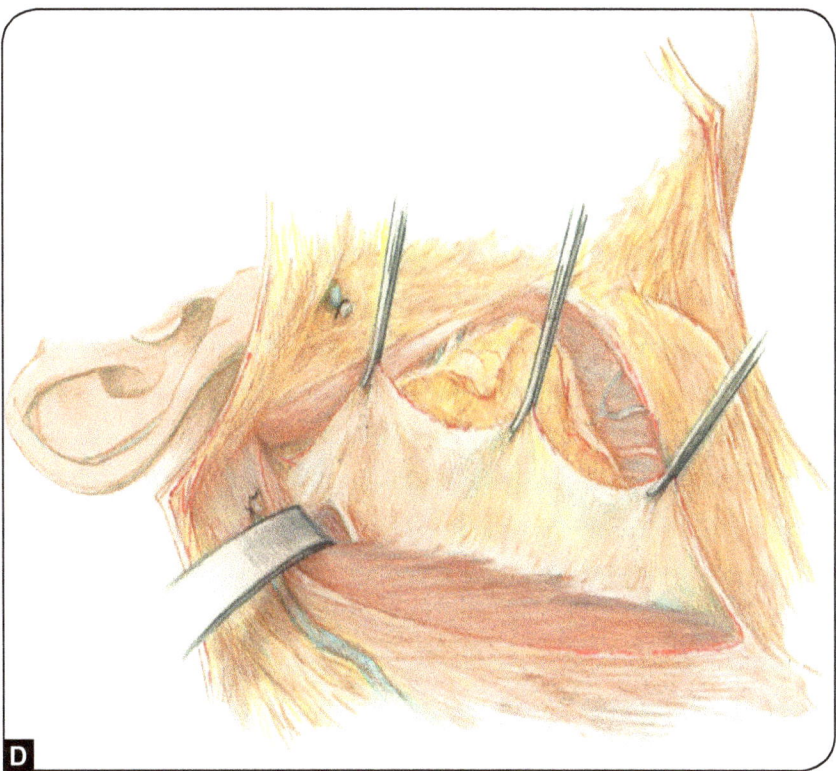

Fig. 1D

- *1E*: Using a mosquito type of hemostat, a fine layer of tissue is elevated over the nerve and it is incised.

- *1F*: It is common to find lymph nodes of various sizes in this area, in this case, anterior to the nerve. The dissection must proceed around these nodes as the fatty tissue lateral to the nerve is incised. Obviously, it is imperative to avoid incising these nodes, as they may contain metastatic tumor.

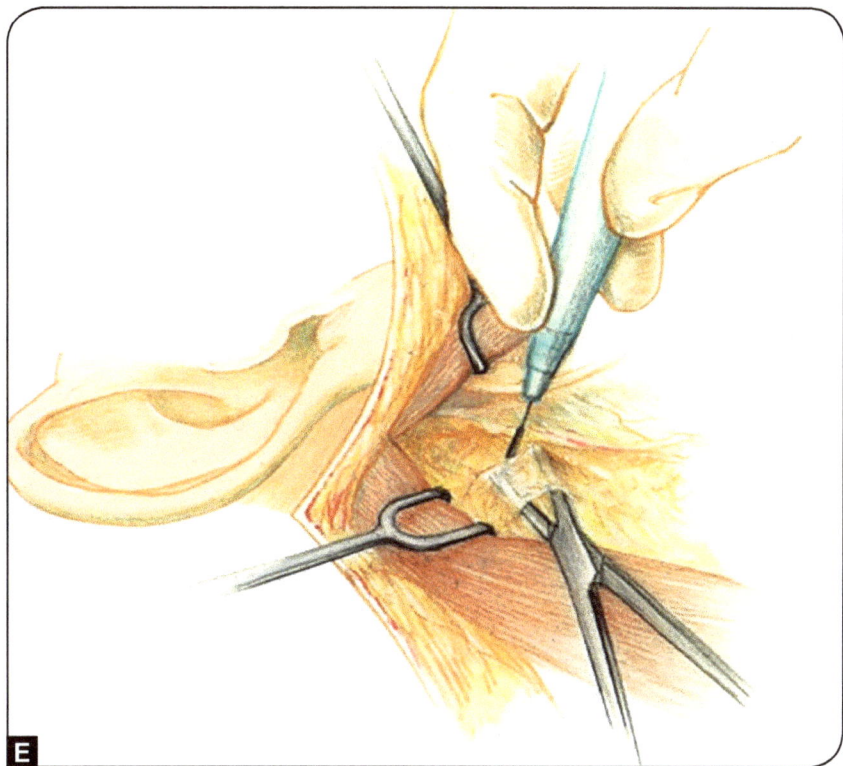

Fig. 1E

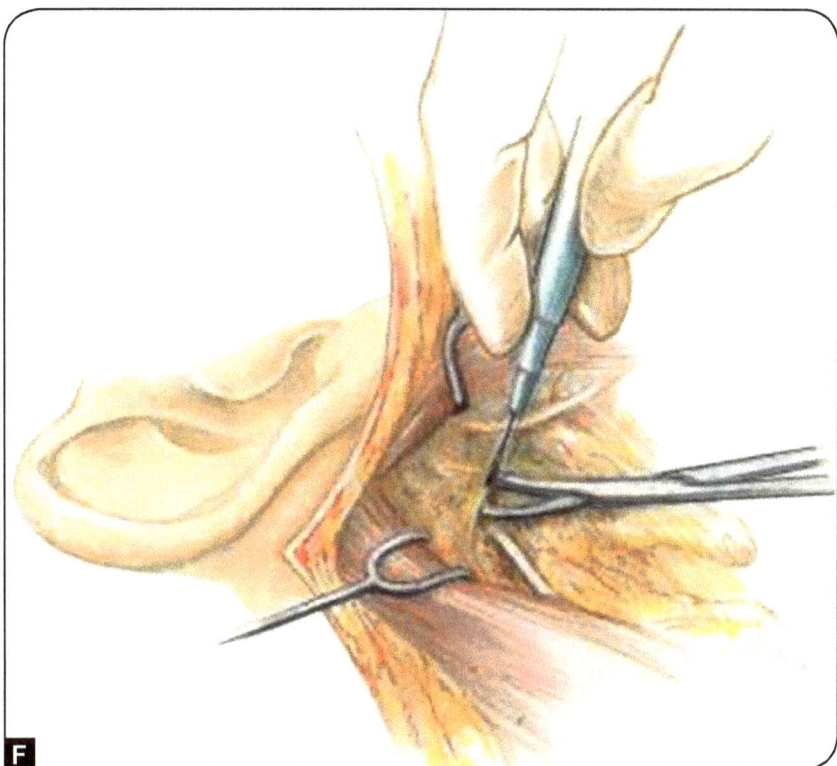

Fig. 1F

- *1G*: The fatty tissue above and behind the spinal accessory nerve is incised along the inferior border of the digastric superiorly and posteriorly, parallel to the posterior border of the SCMM and as far back as possible. Then, the fibro-fatty tissue containing lymph nodes is dissected forward, off the splenius capitis and the levator scapulae muscles.

- *1H*: The dissected tissue from this area of the neck is brought forward under the spinal accessory nerve.

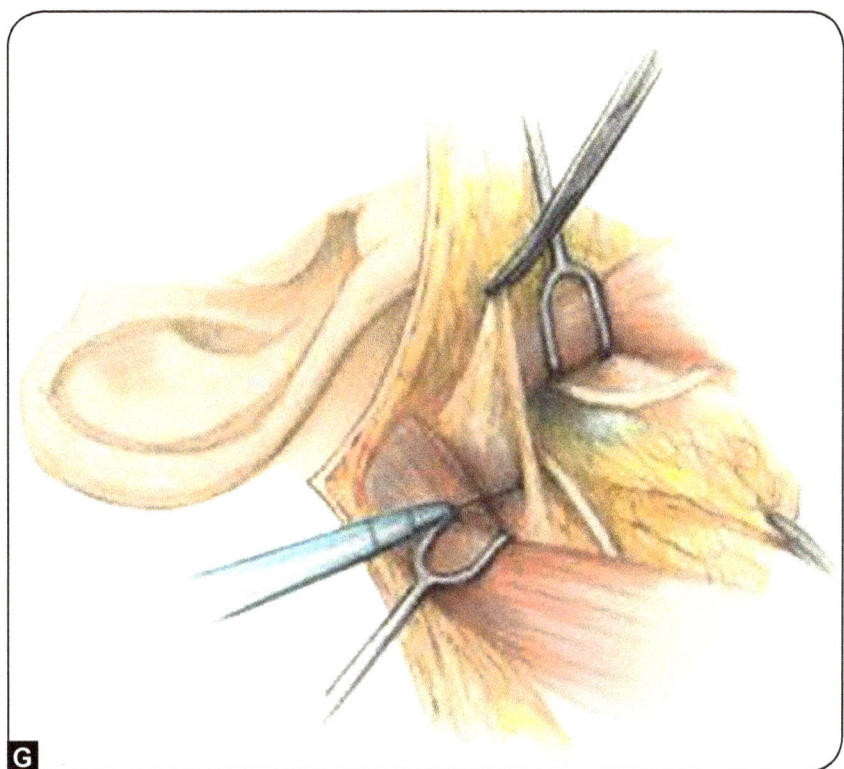

Fig. 1G

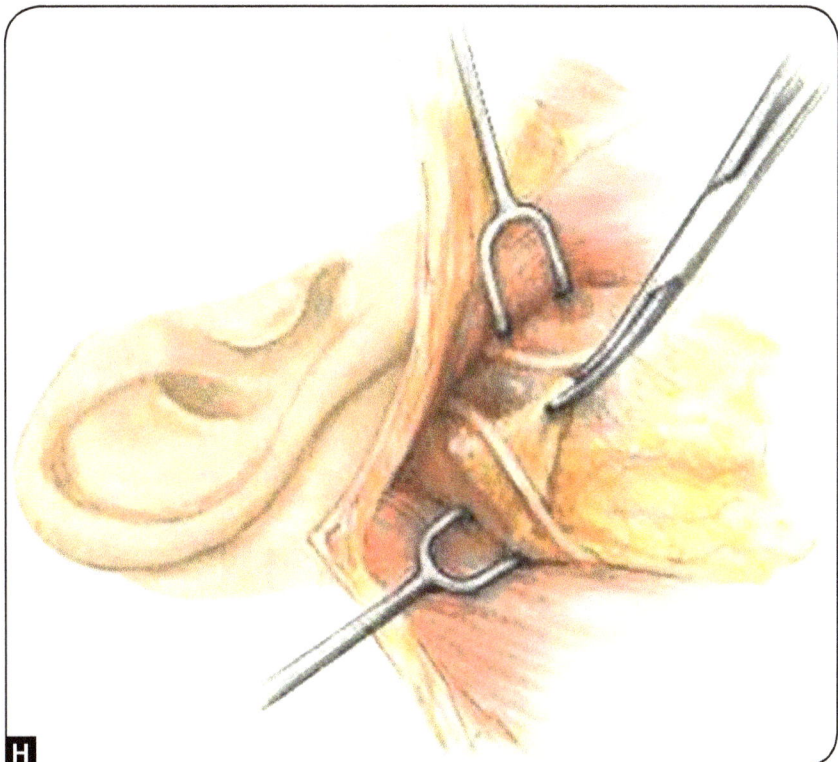

Fig. 1H

Dissection of Level III

Steps of dissection of level III are as follows:

- *2A*: Below the spinal accessory nerve, the posterior limit of the dissection is marked by the cutaneous branches of the cervical plexus, as they reach the posterior border of the SCMM, where they are identified and preserved. To expose these nerves, and depending on the patient's body habitus, a variably thick layer of fatty tissue must be incised in a direction parallel to the posterior border of the SCMM. A safe technique consists of using a fine tip hemostat, such as a mosquito clamp, to pierce the tissue, advance the tip about 1.5 cm in a direction parallel to the posterior border of the SCMM, at a depth of about half a centimeter; then, the hemostat is opened and elevated slightly and the tissue is incised. This is done layer-by-layer until one of the branches of the cervical plexus is exposed. Once this level has been established, the incision of these tissues proceeds downward, more. In this way, a block of adipose tissue containing lymph nodes is formed, which can then be reflected anteriorly.

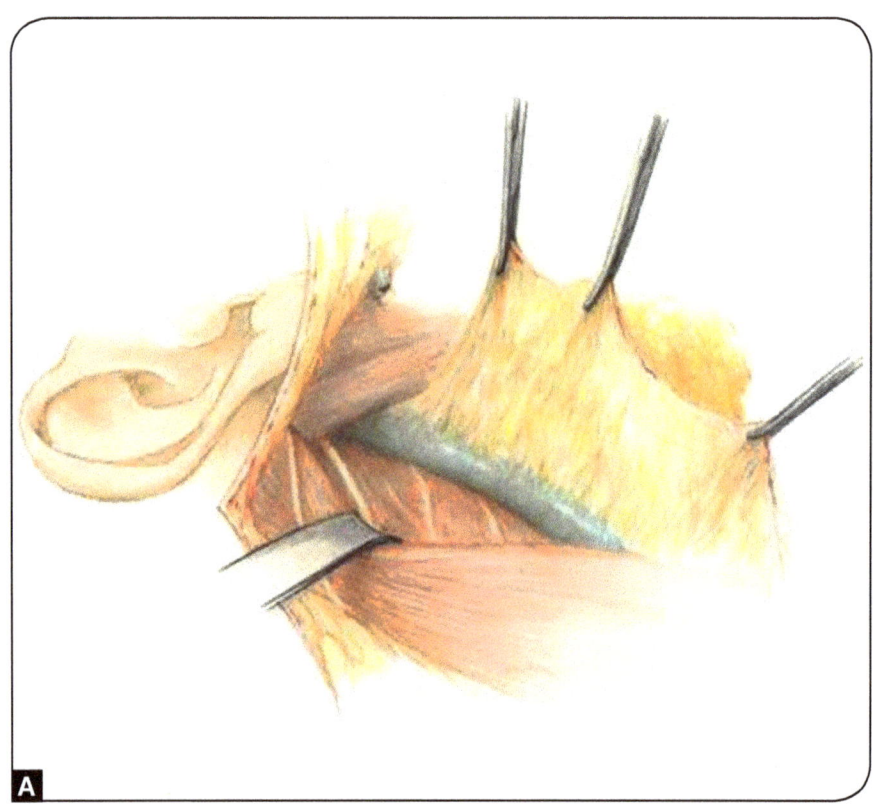

Fig. 2A

Dissection of Level IV

Steps of dissection of level IV are as follows:

- *3A*: Once the level of the omohyoid muscle is reached and this muscle is divided, with the inferior portion of the SCMM maximally retracted laterally, the surgeon can proceed in two ways to safely remove the relatively thick fatty tissue containing lymph nodes in this area.

  In one way, illustrated here, the fascia enveloping the tissue is incised parallel to the clavicle; then, several layers of fascia-like tissue are incised over a hemostat. Eventually, the tissue can be swept upwards exposing a plane immediately lateral to the scalene muscles and the phrenic nerve. Once this plane is established, the tissues can be incised laterally, along or as close to the posterior border of the SCMM as feasible.

  Alternatively, once the level of the omohyoid is reached and the muscle is divided, the fatty tissue below the last exposed cutaneous branch of the cervical plexus is pulled laterally, and the plane lateral to the scalene muscles is identified and entered by means of blunt dissection with a hemostat. When the correct plane is reached, the surgeon can easily insert a finger into the area and bluntly dissect down to the level of the clavicle. Removing the finger and inserting a thin retractor, the phrenic nerve can be visualized; then the thick fatty tissue can be safely incised laterally and then inferiorly.

  In the area of the angle between the clavicle and the IJV, we prefer to clip (using medium or large metal clips) the fatty tissue before incising it. In this way, we occlude small tributaries to the thoracic duct and prevent a chyle leak. The same technique is recommended on both sides of the neck.

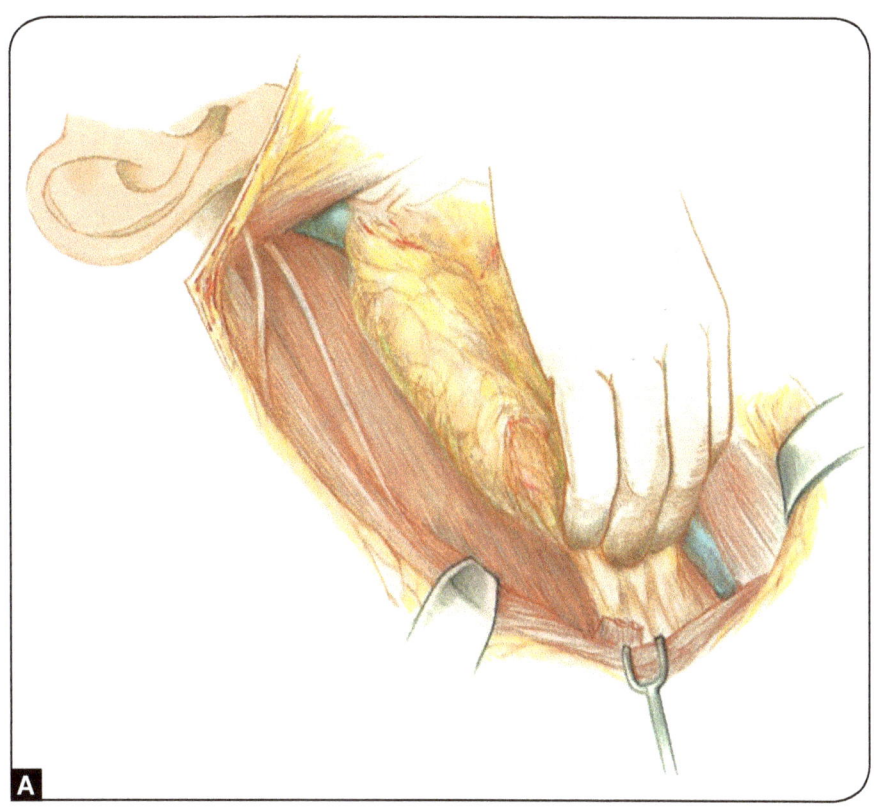

Fig. 3A

- *3B*: The block of fibro-fatty tissue containing lymph nodes from levels II, II and IV is dissected off the cutaneous branches and trunks of the cervical plexus, the levator scapula and the scalene muscles. As the specimen is retracted laterally and forward, the carotid compartment is exposed. The vagus nerve is shown under the hemostat.

- *3C*: The specimen can now be dissected sharply off the IJV. In this case, a superior thyroid branch was divided and ligated.

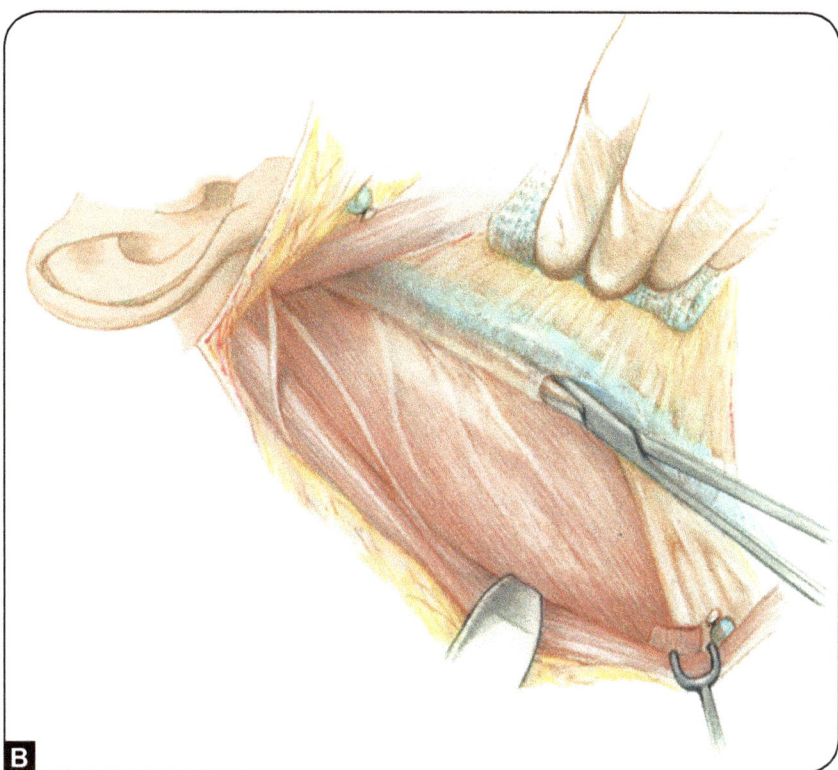

Fig. 3B

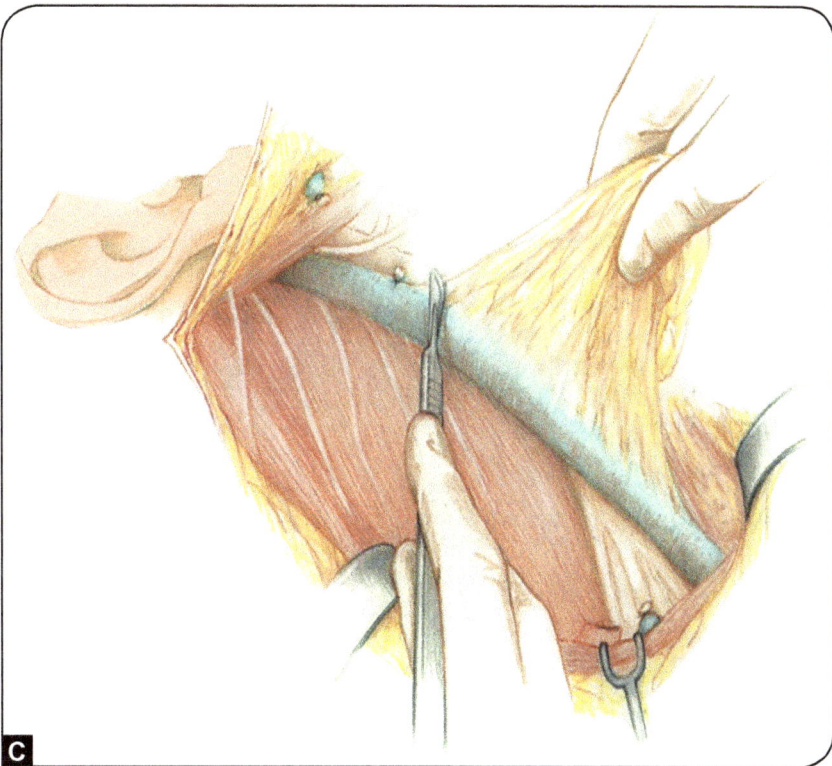

Fig. 3C

- *3D*: Intraoperative photograph showing the relative position of the carotid and vagus nerve.

- *3E*: As the dissection proceeds downwards, the anterior belly of the omohyoid is divided and the specimen is removed.

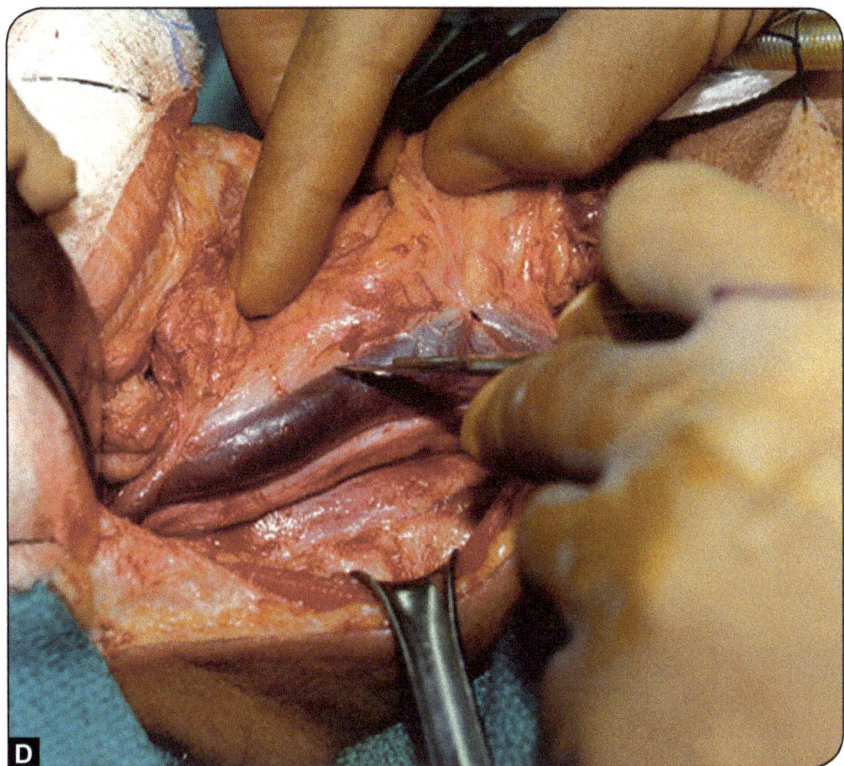

Fig. 3D

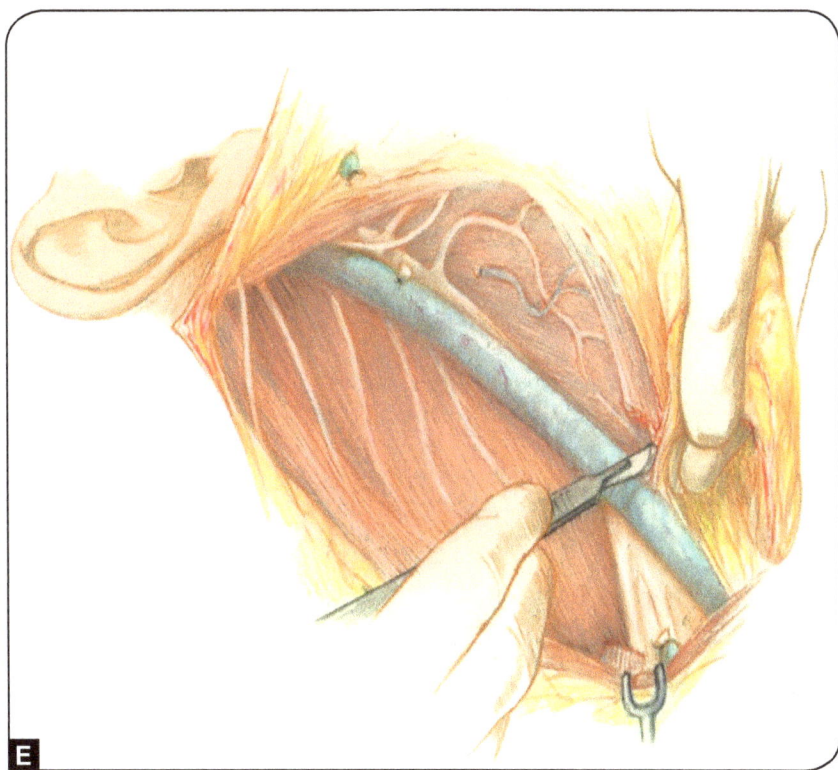

Fig. 3E

■ *3F*: The completed dissection is shown extending from the posterior belly of the digastric superiorly to the clavicle inferiorly, and from the lateral border of the strap muscles anteriorly to the level of the posterior border of the SCMM.

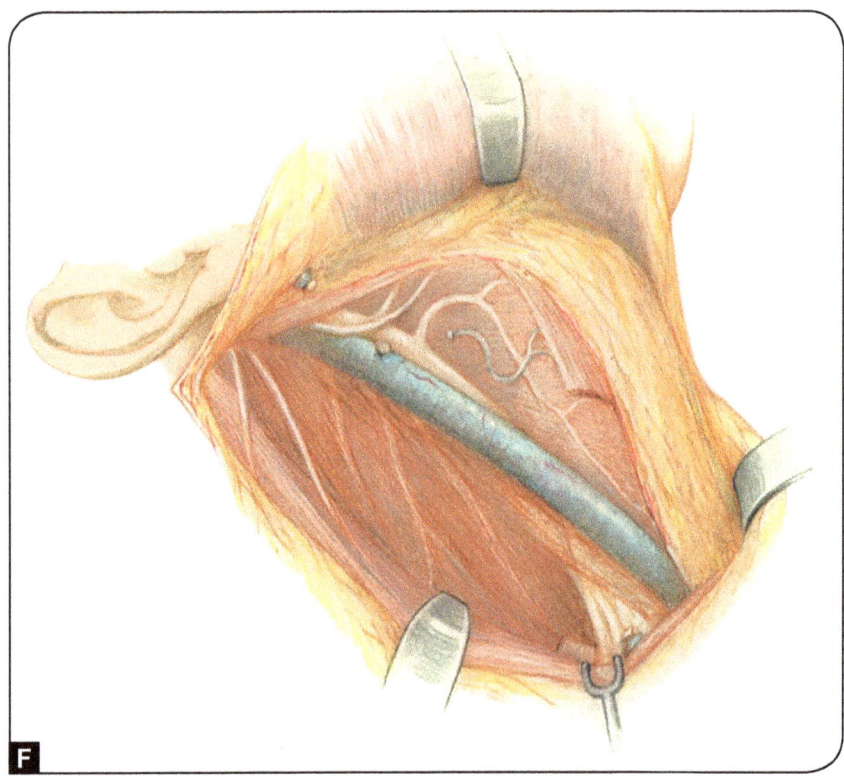

Fig. 3F

REFERENCES

1. Welsh LW. The normal human laryngeal lymphatics. Ann Otol Rhinol Laryngol. 1964;73:569-82.
2. Buckley JG, MacLennan K. Cervical node metastases in laryngeal and hypopharyngeal cancer: a prospective analysis of prevalence and distribution. Head Neck. 2000;22:380-5.
3. Ambrosch P, Freudenberg L, Kron M, Steiner W. Selective neck dissection in the management of squamous cell carcinoma of the upper digestive tract. Eur Arch Otorhinolaryngol. 1996;253(6):329-35.
4. Davidson J, Khan Y, Gilbert R, Birt BD, Balogh J, MacKenzie R. Is selective neck dissection sufficient treatment for the N0/Np+ neck? J. Otolaryngol. 1997;26(4):229-31.
5. Clayman GL, Frank DK. Selective neck dissection of anatomically appropriate levels is as efficacious as modified radical neck dissection for elective treatment of the clinically negative neck in patients with squamous cell carcinoma of the upper respiratory and digestive tracts. Arch Otolaryngol Head Neck Surg. 1998;124(3):348-52.
6. Brazilian Head and Neck Cancer Study Group. End results of a prospective trial on elective lateral neck dissection vs type III modified radical neck dissection in the management of supraglottic and transglottic carcinomas. Head Neck. 1999;21(8):694-702.
7. Ambrosch P, Kron M, Pradier O, et al. Efficacy of selective neck dissection: a review of 503 cases of elective and therapeutic treatment of the neck in squamous cell carcinoma of the upper aerodigestive tract. Otolaryngol Head Neck Surg. 2001;124(2):180-7.
8. Andersen PE, Warren F, Spiro J, et al. Results of selective neck dissection in management of the node-positive neck. Arch Otolaryngol Head Neck Surg. 2002;128(10):1180-4.
9. Robbins KT, Ferlito A, Suarez C, et al. Is there a role for selective neck dissection after chemoradiation for head and neck cancer? J Am Coll Surg. 2004;199(6):913-6.
10. Stenson KM, Haraf DJ, Pelzer H, et al. The role of cervical lymphadenectomy after aggressive concomitant chemoradiotherapy: the feasibility of selective neck dissection. Arch Otolaryngol Head Neck Surg. 2000;126(8):950-6.
11. Medina JE. Cancer of the larynx: Treatment of the neck. In: Fried M, Ferlito A (Eds). The Larynx, Vol II. San Diego: Plural Publishers Inc.; 2009.

CHAPTER 9

Selective Neck Dissection II–V, Suboccipital, Retroauricular (*Posterolateral Neck Dissection*)

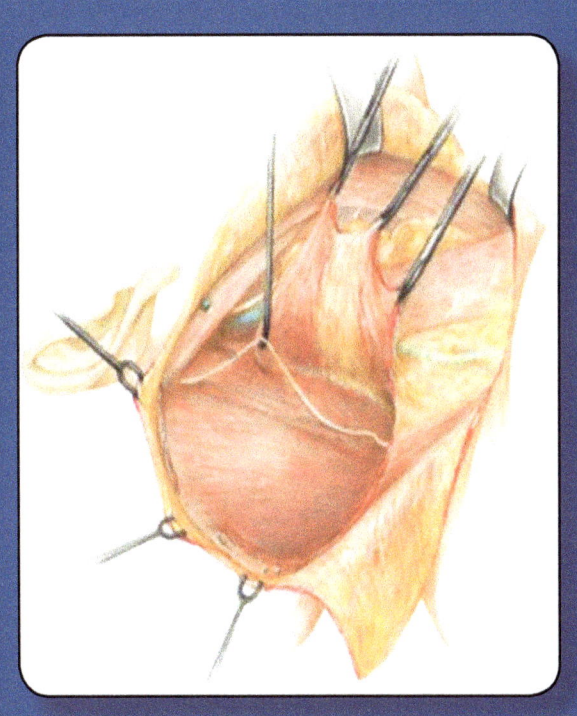

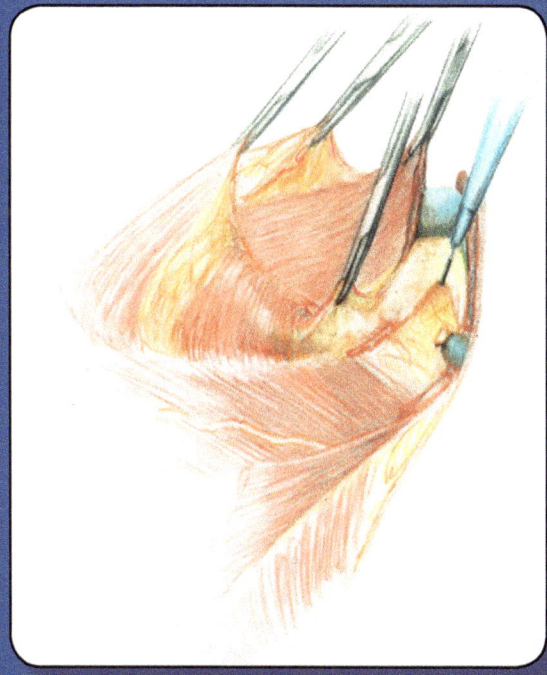

INTRODUCTION

Melanomas of the posterior scalp, posterior superior aspect of the neck and postauricular region metastasize primarily to the retroauricular and suboccipital lymph nodes, which are not included in the standard neck dissections (Fig. 1). These nodes drain into the spinal accessory nodes and also into the upper jugular nodes. Therefore, a therapeutic lymphadenectomy for melanomas in these locations requires a distinct operation that has been named "posterolateral neck dissection". This type of neck dissection was initially described by Rochlin[1] in 1962. It consists of the removal of the suboccipital and retroauricular nodes in addition to the nodes in level II–V. The main variations in surgical technique described in the literature concern the handling of the splenius capitis muscle. Some surgeons describe lymph nodes deep to the upper portion of this muscle, along the deep portion of the occipital artery and advocate resecting it to ensure their removal.[2,3] Most surgeons, however, do not include the splenius in the resection and carry the dissection in a plane immediately superficial to this muscle.[1,4-6] Otherwise, depending on the location and extent of the nodal metastases in the neck, it is often possible to preserve the spinal accessory nerve, the internal jugular vein (IJV) and sometimes the sternocleidomastoid muscle (SCMM).[6]

INDICATIONS

A posterolateral neck dissection is indicated in the treatment of clinically evident lymph node metastases from melanomas, squamous cell carcinomas, or Merkel cell carcinomas that originate in the posterior and posterolateral aspects of the neck and the scalp.

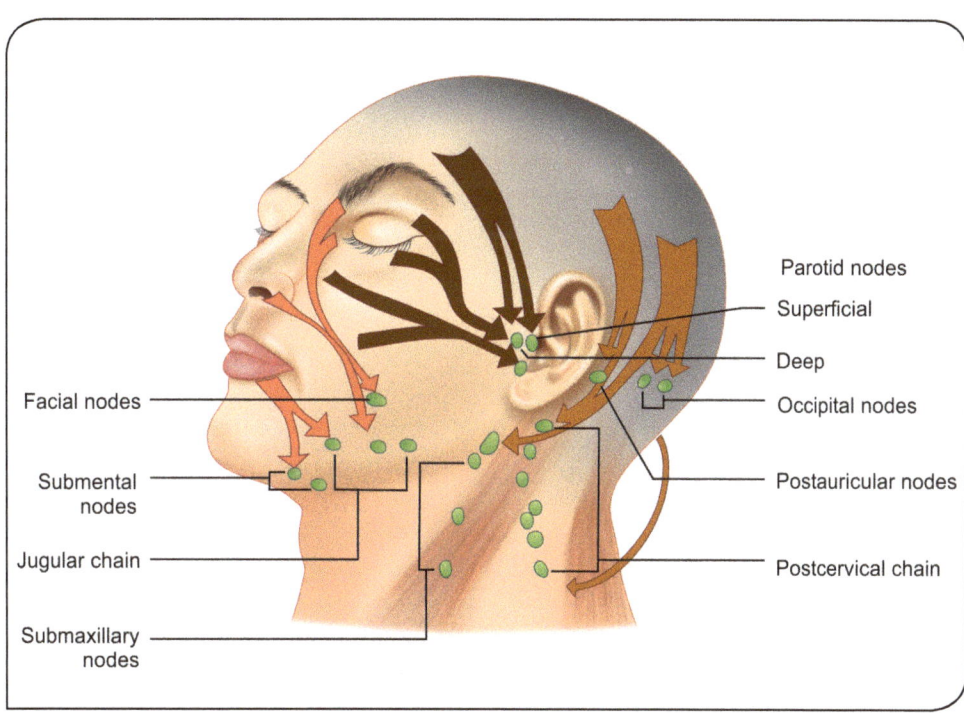

Fig. 1: Lymphatic drainage of the face and scalp.

SURGICAL TECHNIQUE

■ *2A*: A unilateral posterolateral neck dissection is performed by placing the patient in the supine position with a beanbag under the chest and shoulders and the head on a horseshoe head holder. Alternatively, a tall donut-shaped sponge may be used to support the head, which is turned away from the side of the neck to be dissected. When a bilateral dissection is to be performed, the patient must be placed in the prone position with the head slightly flexed downward.
The incision commonly used to perform a posterolateral neck dissection is shaped like a hockey stick, with a horizontal portion placed at the level of the nuchal line. The vertical portion of it is placed between the posterior border of the SCMM and the anterior border of the trapezius, and its direction parallels the latter; it curves forward about two finger breaths above the clavicle.

■ *2B*: Frequently, the incision around the primary melanoma has to be blended with neck incision, as it is shown in this intraoperative photograph.

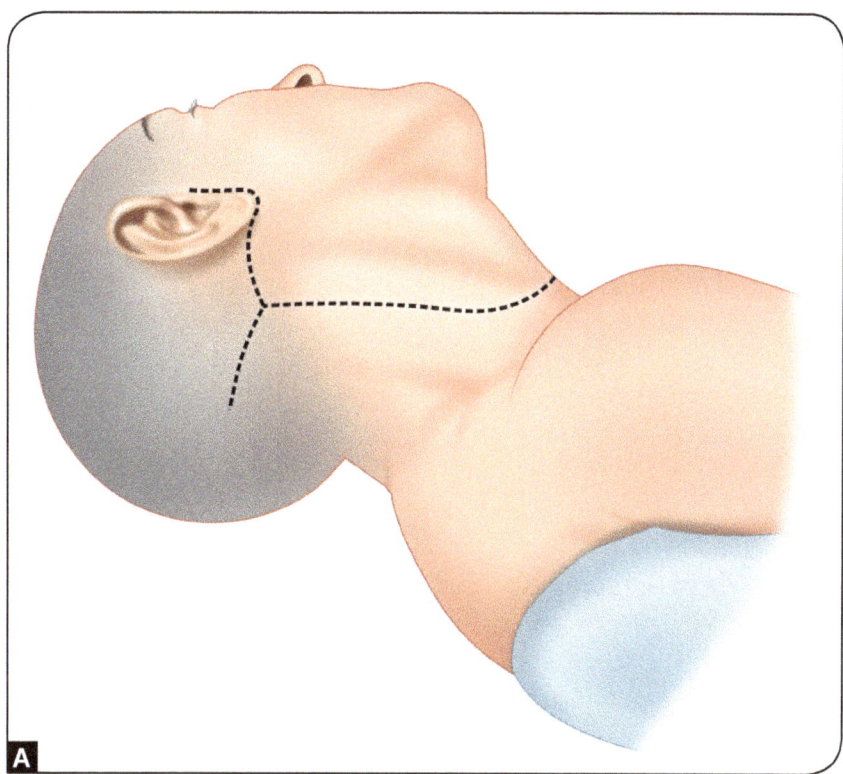

Fig. 2A

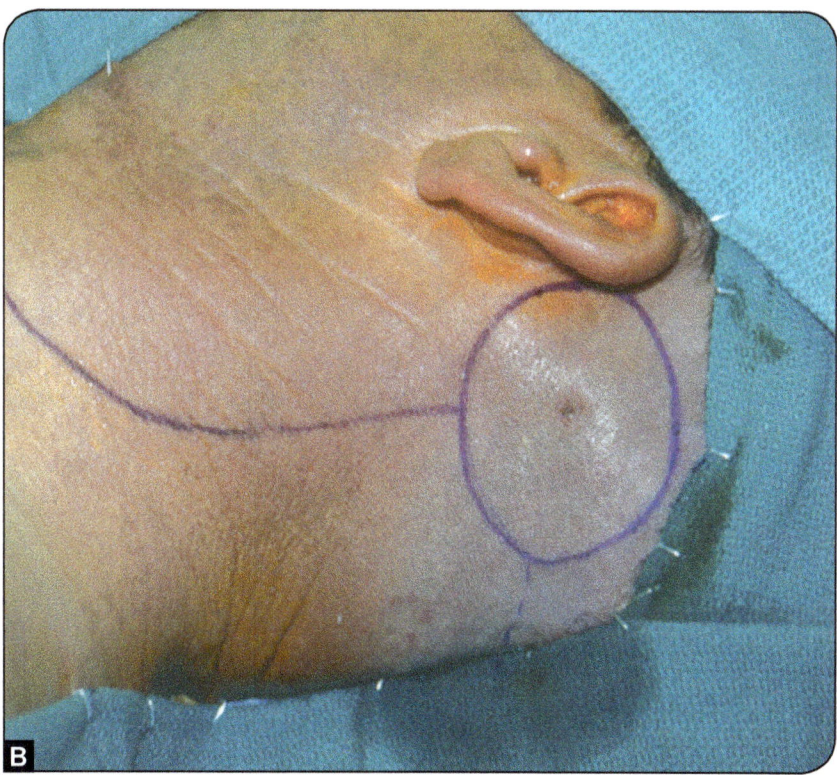

Fig. 2B

- *2C*: A unique step in this operation is the elevation of the posterior skin flap, which must extend to the posterior midline of the neck in a superficial subcutaneous plane. Unfortunately, there is no anatomic plane to help define the proper thickness of this flap, which is crucial; if the flap is too thin, the anterior portion of it may necrose; on the other hand, if the flap is too thick, some of the suboccipital nodes, which are very superficial, may be elevated with it, defeating the purpose of the operation. The anterior flap is elevated until the anterior border of the SCMM is reached.

  The spinal accessory nerve is identified early in the dissection and it is exposed throughout its course in the neck. To review the different ways to identify the nerve in the posterior triangle of the neck, the reader is referred to the Chapter 6, Section entitled Dissection of the Spinal Accessory: 1A-1C.

  In this illustration, the nerve is initially exposed in front of the anterior border of the trapezius muscle. With the help of a hemostat, the thin tissue covering the nerve is elevated and incised.

- *2D*: With the nerve under direct vision, the fibers of the SCMM overlying are divided. The nerve has been exposed in its entirety and is then freed from the surrounding tissues throughout its course between the trapezius and the posterior belly of the digastric muscle.

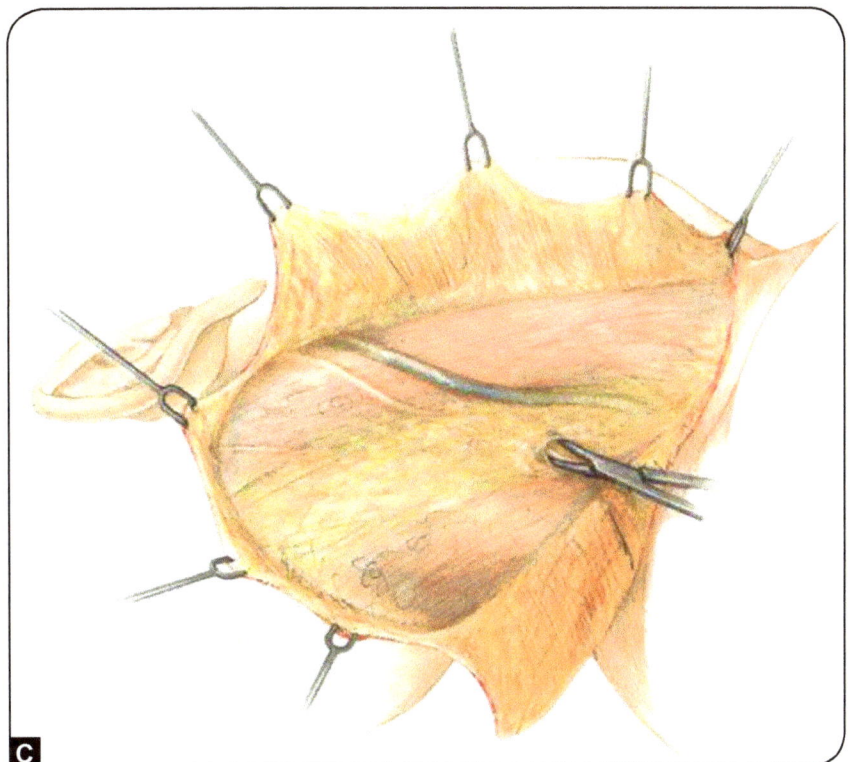

Fig. 2C

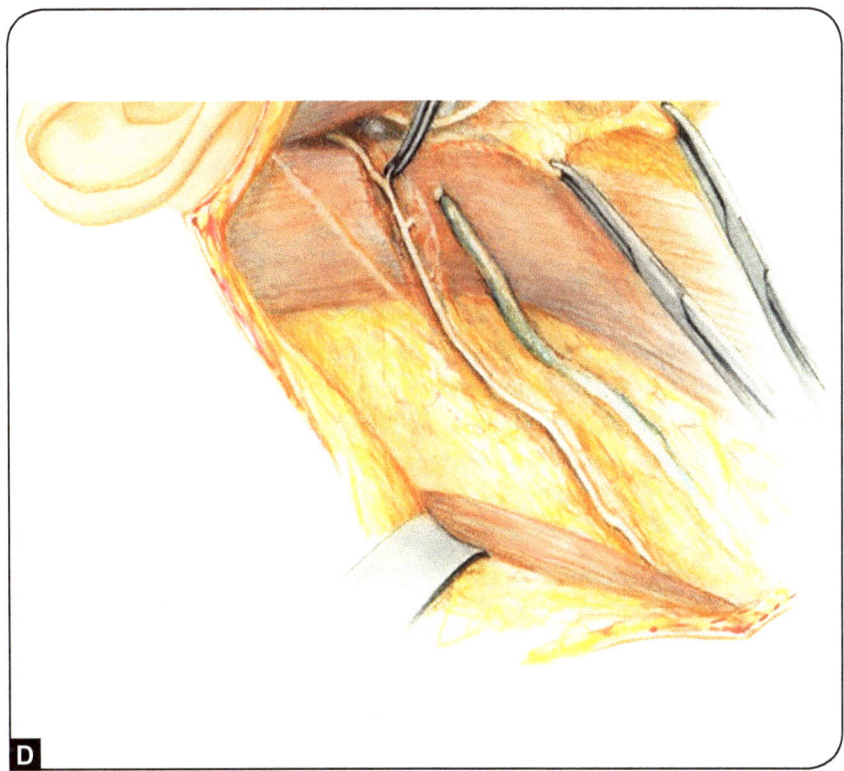

Fig. 2D

- *2E*: The dissection begins by incising the fatty tissue overlying the trapezius and the trapezius muscle itself, above the level of the spinal accessory nerve. This incision is made obliquely upwards and towards the posterior midline. In the depth, the aim is to reach the plane immediately superficial to the splenius capitis muscle. Identification of this plane is easier low in the neck and then the incision continues upward and backward toward the posterior midline of the neck at the nuchal line.

- *2F*: The superior tendinous insertion of the trapezius is incised along the nuchal line. As this is done, from medial to lateral, the greater occipital nerve and the occipital artery are identified and divided. The greater occipital nerve becomes superficial just inferior to the superior nuchal line, about a third of the way between the posterior midline and the mastoid or about 4 cm lateral to the external occipital protuberance. At this point, the nerve is positioned medial to the occipital artery.

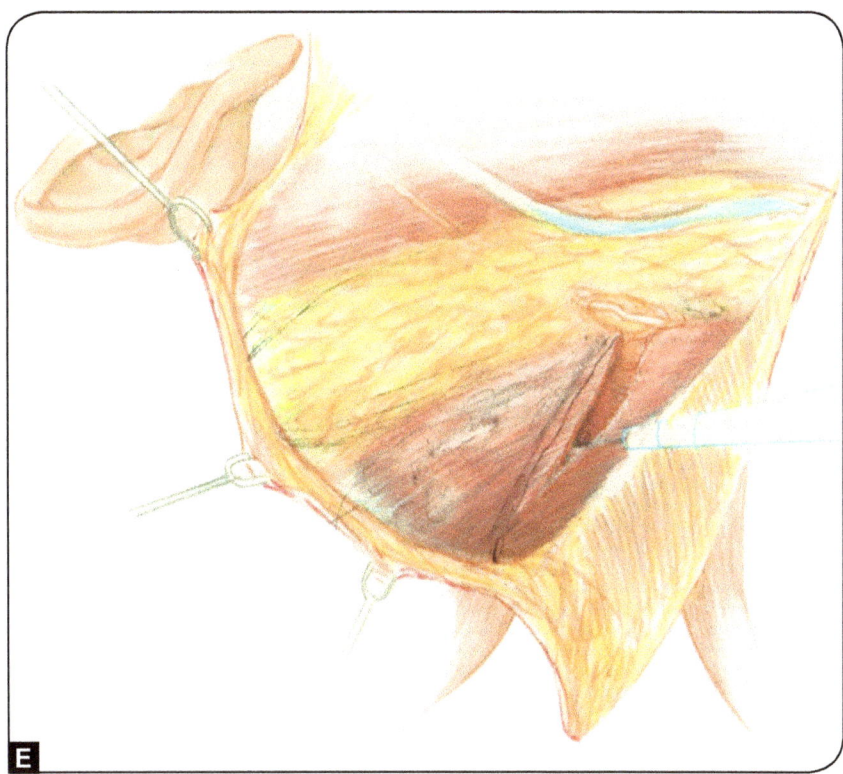

Fig. 2E

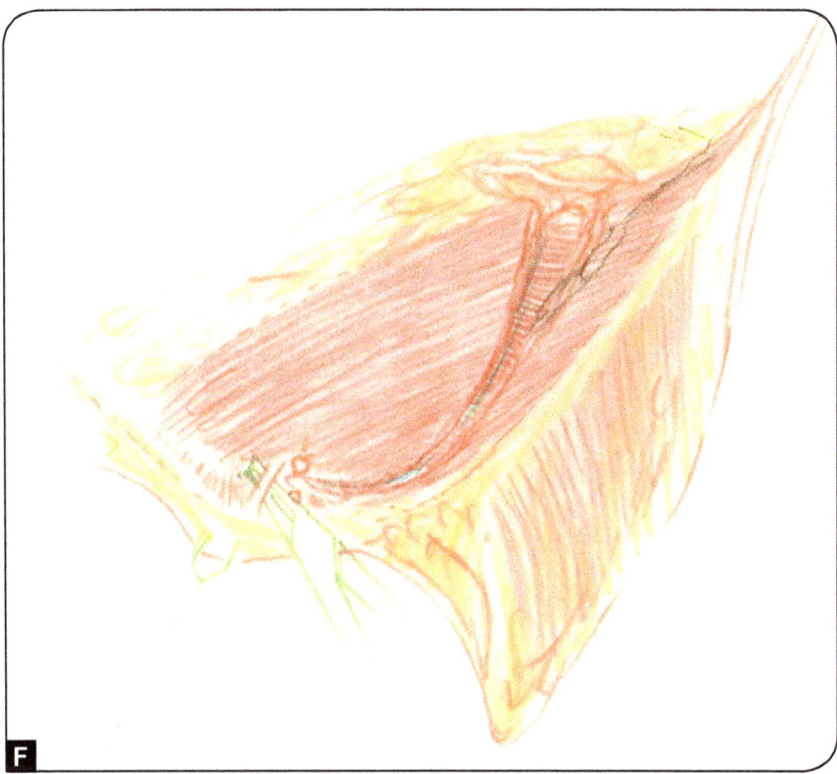

Fig. 2F

- *2G*: The division of the superior insertion of the trapezius and the SCMM continues laterally. While in this illustration, it is shown as a separate step, this incision is usually carried out as the specimen is dissected forward and downward in the plane immediately superficial to the splenius capitis, as it is shown in Figure 2G. Doing the operation in this manner prevents inadvertent incision of the upper insertions of the splenius capitis, which is otherwise easy to do because the superior ends of the trapezius and the splenius fuse into a common tendinous structure near the nuchal line.

  Alternatively, the trapezius muscle is not incised at all and the fascia and fibro-fatty tissue over and under its superior portion is dissected off of it.

- *2H*: As the dissection proceeds forward, the plane of dissection changes from the splenius capitis to the levator scapulae. Superiorly, the retroauricular lymph node or nodes are included in the specimen, and the superior insertion of the SCMM is incised near the mastoid process.

  When the specimen is freed enough, it is brought forward under the spinal accessory nerve if it is being preserved. Below the posterior belly of the digastric, the upper end of the IJV and the hypoglossal nerve are exposed and preserved.

  Alternatively, the SCMM is preserved and the retroauricular tissue containing lymph nodes is dissected from it. Instead of transecting the muscle, the fascia and fibro-fatty tissue enveloping it is dissected from it circumferentially, as it is described in Chapter 5.

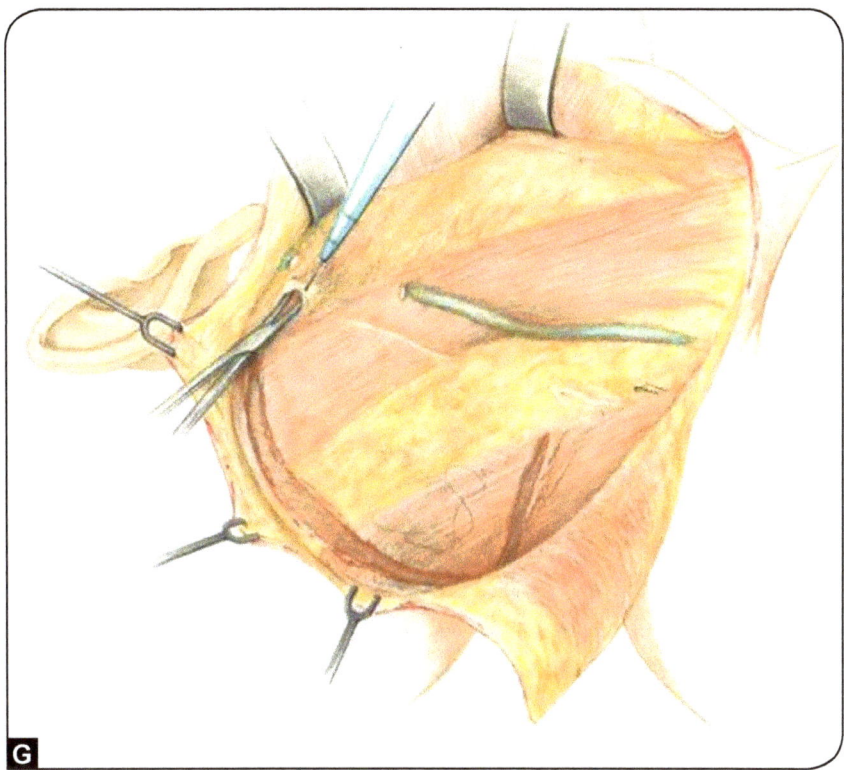

Fig. 2G

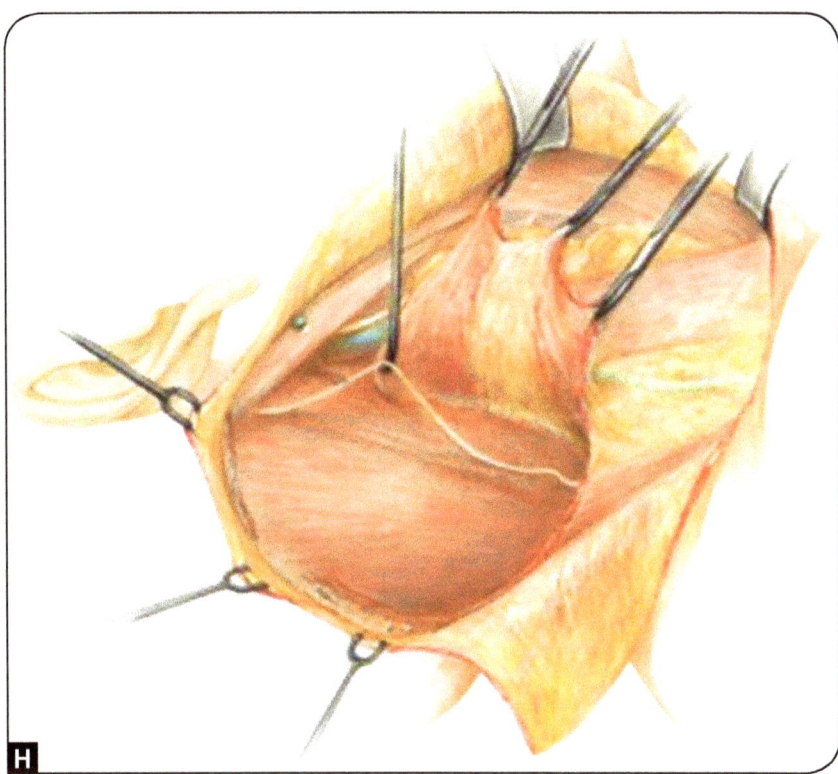

Fig. 2H

- *2I*: The dissection continues downward and medially, above the clavicle. The inferior insertion of the SCMM, the branches of the cervical plexus and the external jugular vein are divided. The inferior most portion of the IJV is exposed. Depending on the characteristics of the tumor in the neck, it is often possible to preserve the IJV. Then, the fascia and adipose between the IJV and the anterior border of the trapezius are incised layer-by-layer; the posterior belly of the omohyoid muscle is divided. Eventually, the fibro-fatty tissue above the clavicle can be swept upward exposing the brachial plexus and the phrenic nerve.

- *2J*: The specimen is dissected off of the levator scapula, the levator scapula and the scalene muscles, preserving the nerves to the levator as described in Chapter 3, Section entitled Dissection of the Posterior Triangle. Then, it is sharply dissected from the IJV. As the dissection proceeds superiorly, an anterior facial vein is divided below the hypoglossal nerve to free the specimen.

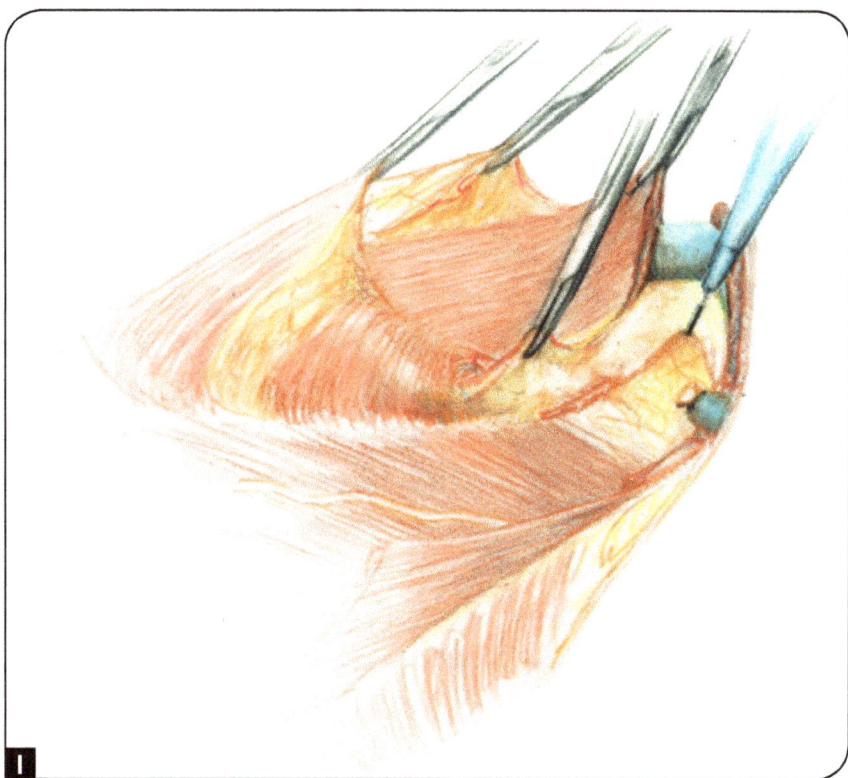

Fig. 2I

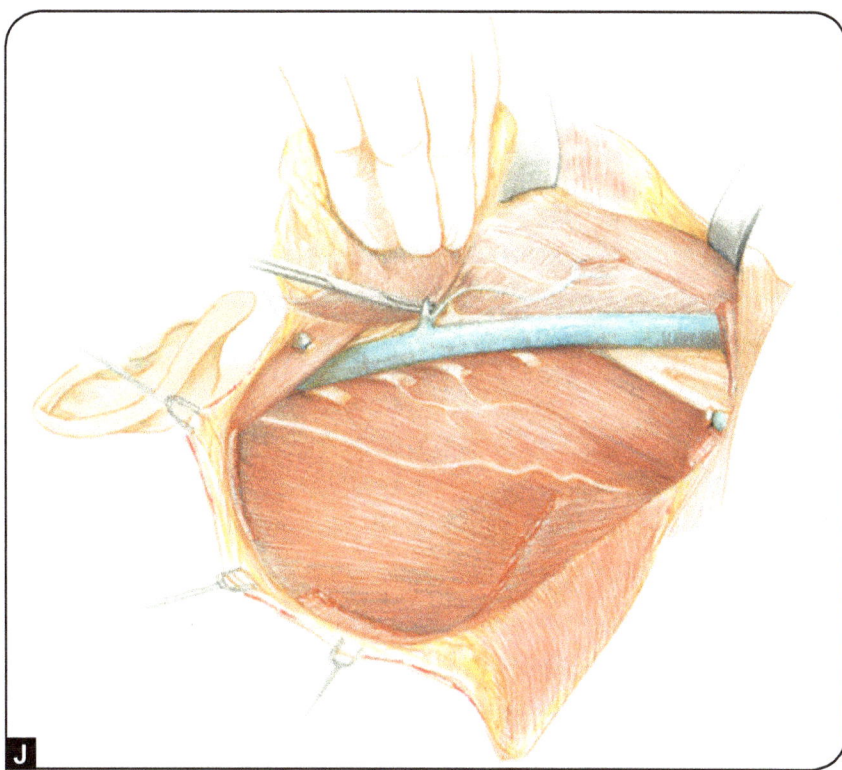

Fig. 2J

- *2K*: The completed dissection is shown extending from the nuchal line superiorly to the clavicle inferiorly, and from the posterior midline posterior-superiorly to the lateral border of the strap muscles anteriorly.

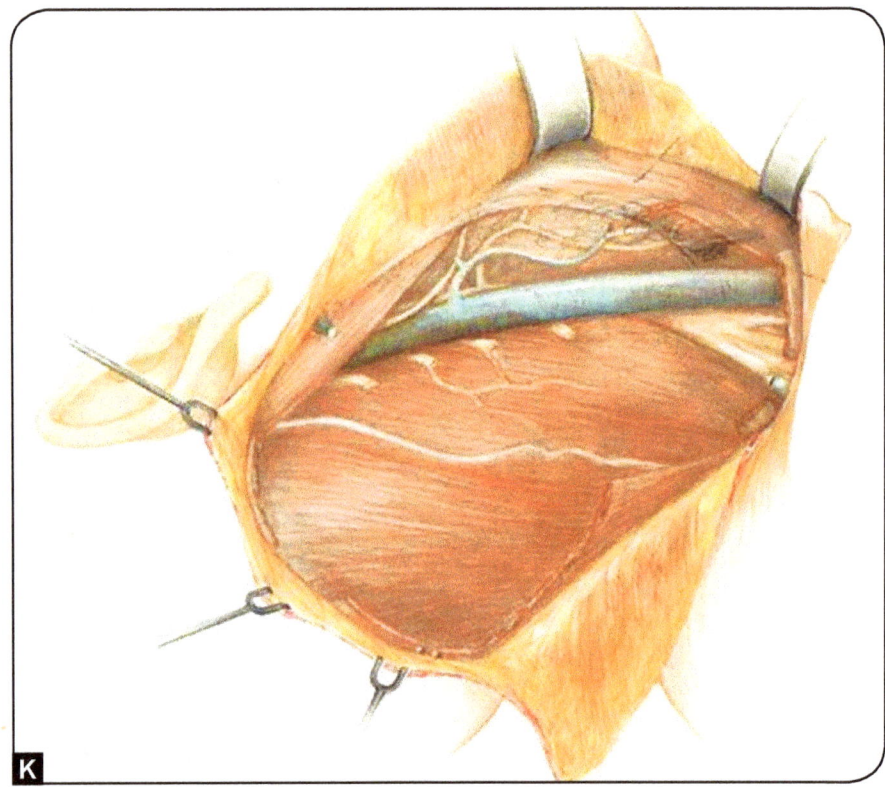

Figs. 2A to K: Posterolateral neck dissection.

REFERENCES

1. Rochlin DB. Posterolateral neck dissection for malignant neoplasms. Surg Gynecol Obstet. 1962;115:369-73.
2. Wander JV, Chaudhuri PK. Dissection of the posterior part of the neck. Surg Gynecol Obstet. 1976;143(1):97-100.
3. Fisher SR, Cole TB, Seigler HF. Application of posterior neck dissection in treating malignant melanoma of the posterior scalp. Laryngoscope. 1983;93(6):760-5.
4. Goepfert H, Jesse RH, Ballantyne AJ. Posterolateral neck dissection. Arch Otolaryngol. 1980;106(10):618-20.
5. de Langen ZJ, Vermey A. Posterolateral neck dissection. Head Neck Surg. 1988;10(4):252-6.
6. Medina JE. Posterolateral neck dissection. Oper Tech Otolaryngol Head Neck Surg. 2004;15(3):176-9.

CHAPTER 10

Selective Neck Dissection of Level VI
(Central Compartment Dissection)

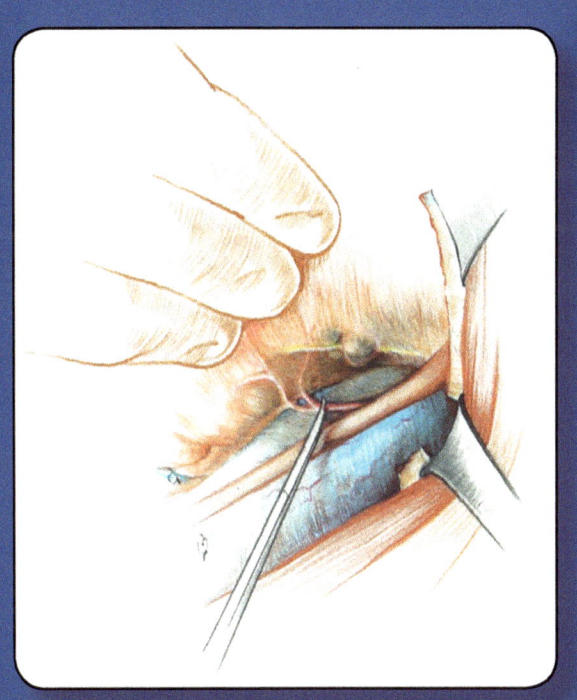
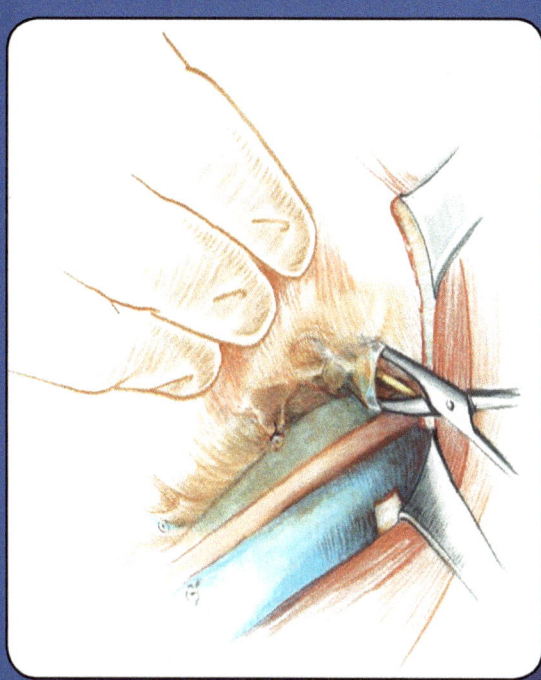

INTRODUCTION

The central compartment of the neck, also referred to as the anterior compartment of the neck or cervical lymph node level VI, is defined in the classification of neck node levels of the American Academy of Otolaryngology-Head and Neck Surgery (AAOHNS) as the compartment of the neck that includes the precricoid (Delphian), pretracheal, paratracheal, and perithyroidal nodes, including the nodes along the recurrent laryngeal nerves.[1] The superior boundary of this compartment is the hyoid bone, the inferior boundary is the suprasternal notch and the lateral boundaries are the common carotid arteries. These boundaries have also been defined radiologically by Som et al.[2]

Several classical studies of the distribution of lymphatics of the different areas of the larynx have shown that efferent lymphatics from the subglottic region terminate in the paratracheal lymph nodes or in the prelaryngeal and pretracheal nodes.[3] In addition, posterolateral lymphatic pedicles (three to six in number), some of which originate in the laryngeal ventricle exit the larynx through the cricotracheal membrane and terminate in the more superior paratracheal nodes.[4,5]

The lymphatics from the inferior-medial aspect of the thyroid lobes follow the course of the inferior thyroid veins and drain to pretracheal, paratracheal (level VI) and lower jugular lymph nodes (level IV). They drain secondarily into the nodes of the anterior-superior mediastinum (level VII) and rarely into lower mediastinal nodes. The lymphatics emerging from the lateral and superior aspects of the gland drain into the nodes in levels III, IV and II.

Lymph node metastases from thyroid carcinoma tend to occur first in the paratracheal nodes regardless of the location of the primary within the thyroid gland.[6,7] A sentinel lymph node from the thyroid can be detected in the paratracheal region in 88% of the patients.[8]

INDICATIONS

Dissection of the nodes in the central compartment of the neck is indicated in the following situations.

Carcinomas of the Thyroid

Papillary Carcinoma

The role of elective dissection of the lymph nodes in the central compartment of the neck is the main controversy in the surgical management of differentiated carcinoma of the thyroid today.[10] The most recent guidelines published by the American Thyroid Association[11] state that "prophylactic central compartment neck dissection (ipsilateral or bilateral)" may be performed in patients with papillary thyroid carcinoma with clinically uninvolved central neck lymph nodes, especially for advanced primary tumors (T3 or T4).

Medullary Carcinoma

Elective central compartment (level VI) neck dissection is indicated in patients with no evidence of advanced local invasion by the primary tumor, no evidence of cervical lymph node metastases on physical examination and cervical ultrasound (US), and no evidence of distant metastases.[12]

It is also indicated when there is clinical or imaging evidence of metastases to the nodes of the central compartment.

Carcinoma of the Larynx

When the following tumors of the larynx are treated surgically, particularly, when the tumor is persistent or recurrent after previous treatment with radiation with or without chemotherapy.[9]

- *Primary subglottic carcinomas*: Dissection in these cases should include the pretracheal and the paratracheal nodes on both sides.
- Advanced (T3–T4) glottic carcinomas particularly those with involvement of the anterior commissure and with subglottic extension. In tumors confined to one side of the larynx, treatment or dissection should include the prelaryngeal, pretracheal and the ipsilateral paratracheal nodes. In tumors involving both sides of the larynx, treatment should include the paratracheal nodes on both sides.
- Advanced (T3–T4) supraglottic carcinomas, particularly those with involvement of the ventricle or paraglottic space, the anterior commissure and those with clinically apparent lymph node metastases in the lateral compartment of the neck. In tumors confined to one side of the larynx, treatment or dissection should include the prelarygneal, pretracheal and the ipsilateral paratracheal nodes. In tumors involving both sides of the larynx, treatment should include the paratracheal nodes on both sides.

SURGICAL TECHNIQUE

The central compartment dissection may be performed with or without a neck dissection. It can be done before or after the neck dissection is completed. It also differs depending on whether the operation is done for cancer of the thyroid or for cancer of the larynx in conjunction with a total laryngectomy.

With Thyroidectomy

- *1A*: Once the neck dissection is completed and the internal jugular vein (IJV) is exposed, the dissection moves on to the anterior and medial aspects of the common carotid artery. In this process, the middle thyroid vein is divided between clamps and ligated.

- *1B*: The dissection is carried inferiorly in the mostly avascular plane medial to the common carotid. The omohyoid muscle or its intermediate tendon is divided. Depending upon the anterior extent of the tumor in the thyroid, the sternohyoid muscle may be retracted or may be transected. In the case illustrated here, the sternohyoid and the sternothyroid muscles are divided from lateral to medial, immediately above the clavicle and the suprasternal notch.

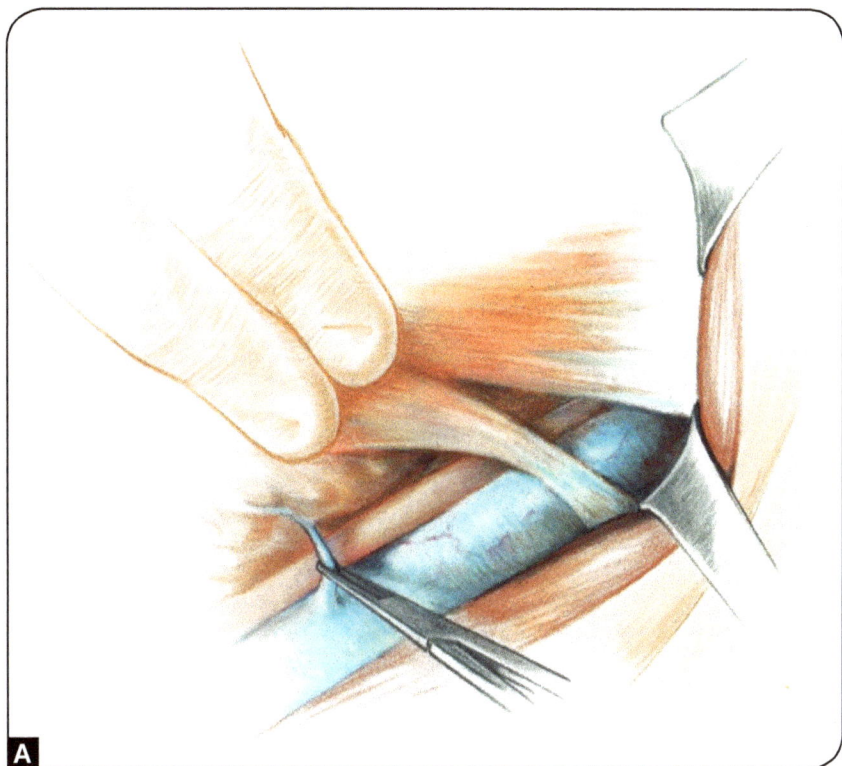

Fig. 1A

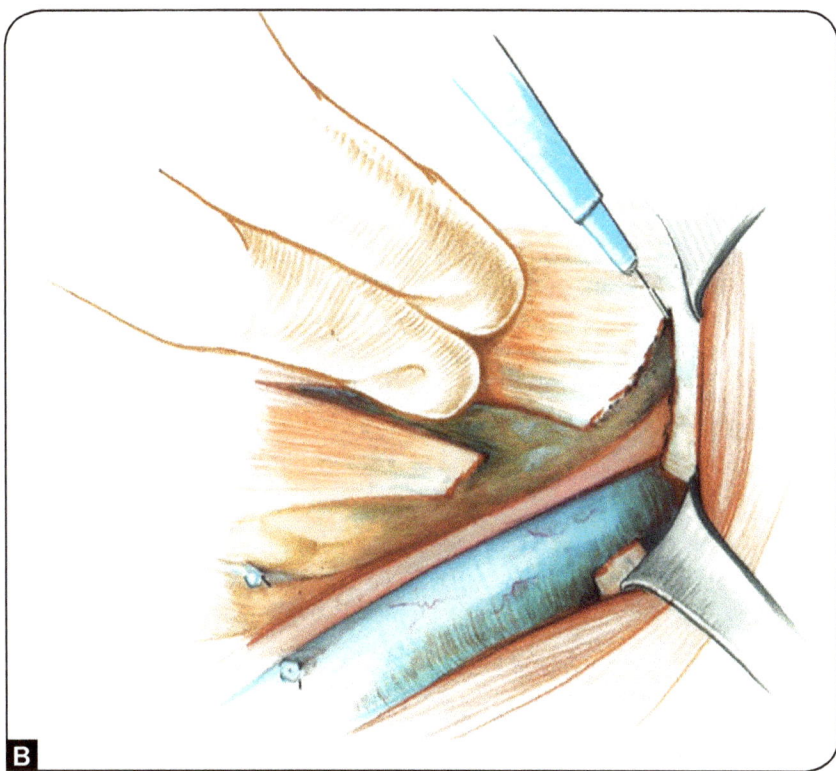

Fig. 1B

- *1C*: The common carotid artery may need to be retracted gently to expose the inferior thyroid artery. Whenever possible, the main trunk of this artery is preserved and the distal branches are dissected. This may lead to the identification of the inferior parathyroid gland, which can then be dissected free and preserved. If the inferior parathyroid is not identified, an effort is made to ligate only the lower most branches of the artery, as the upper branches may supply the superior parathyroid gland.

- *1D*: The dissection continues along the medial aspect of the right common carotid artery up to the level of the innominate artery. Then, the fibro-fatty tissue anterior to the trachea, and in some instances remnants of the thymus, are divided in a layer-by-layer manner. Care is taken to expose and ligate the inferior thyroid veins. On the right side, the recurrent laryngeal nerve is identified as it courses superiorly from lateral to medial, deep to the innominate artery, medial to the common carotid and variably lateral to the tracheoesophageal groove. On the left side, the nerve is closer to the tracheoesophageal groove. Using a hemostat to elevate the tissues over it, the nerve is exposed and freed up from inferior to superior.

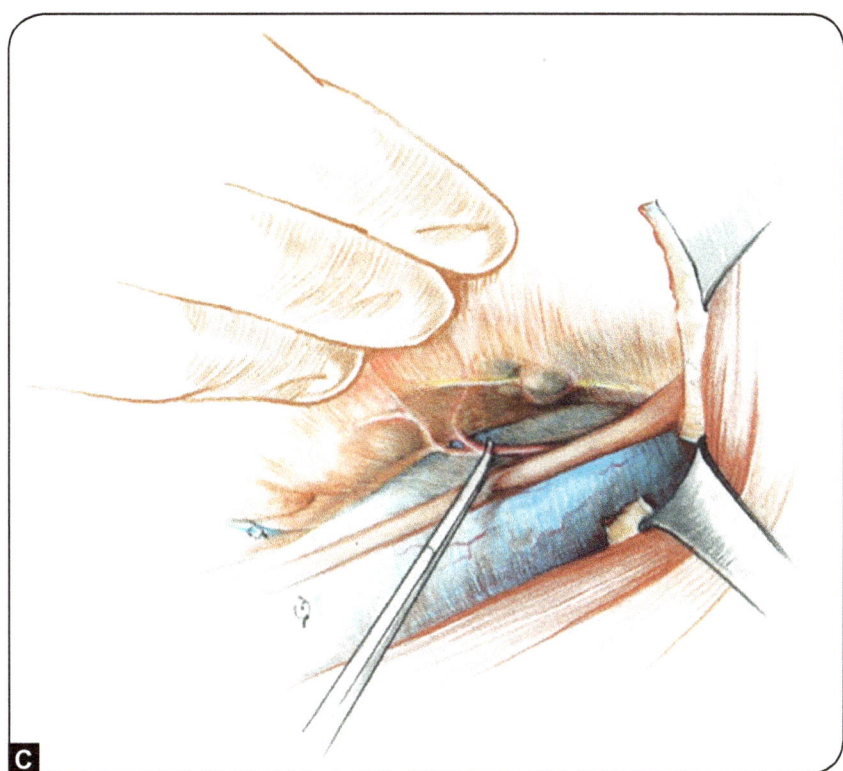

Fig. 1C

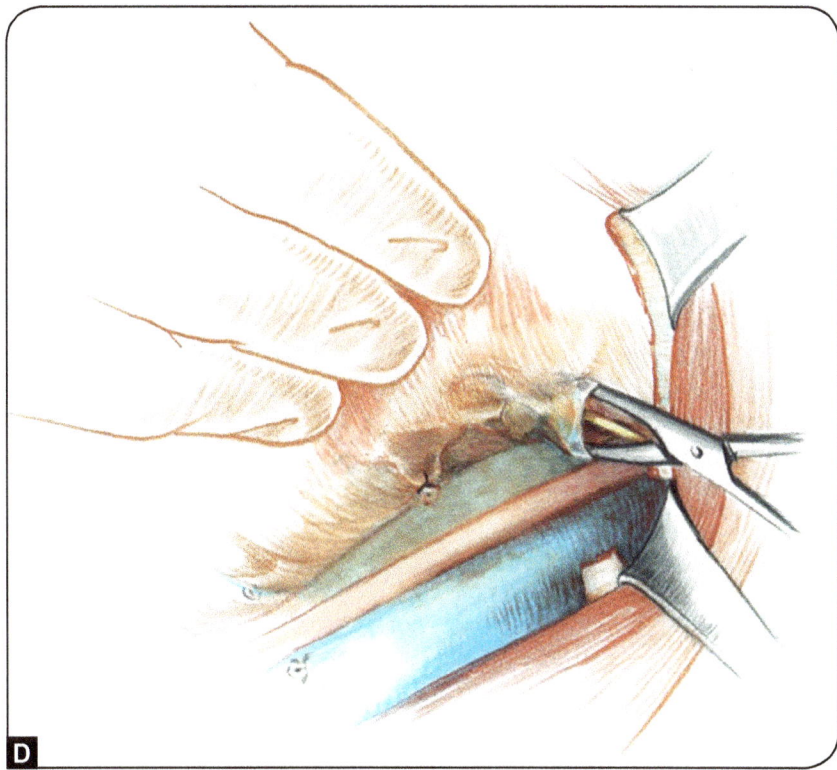

Fig. 1D

- *1E*: Then, the fatty tissue and lymph nodes are dissected off of the esophagus, the tracheoesophageal groove, and the lateral and anterior tracheal walls. During this part of the dissection, it is useful to coagulate the fatty areolar tissue with a bipolar forceps before cutting it, in order to maintain a bloodless field.

- *1F*: Alternatively, and particularly when the dissection is done electively or when paratracheal nodes involved with tumor are not in close proximity to the thyroid, the thyroid lobe is removed up to the point where only its anterior attachments to the trachea remain. Grabbing the lobe attached to the trachea facilitates retraction of the trachea superiorly and provides the needed exposure of the tracheoesophageal area. Since, the recurrent laryngeal nerve has already been exposed superiorly, it is freed up from superior to inferior and, then, the paratracheal and pretracheal fibro-fattty tissue and lymph nodes are dissected off the trachea, esophagus and tracheoesophageal groove.

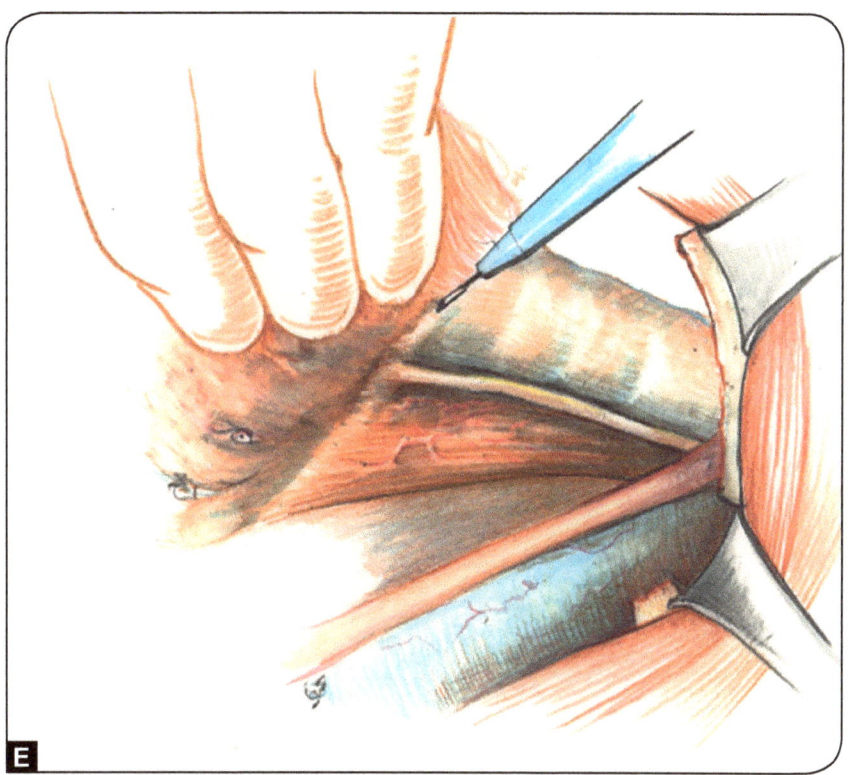

Fig. 1E

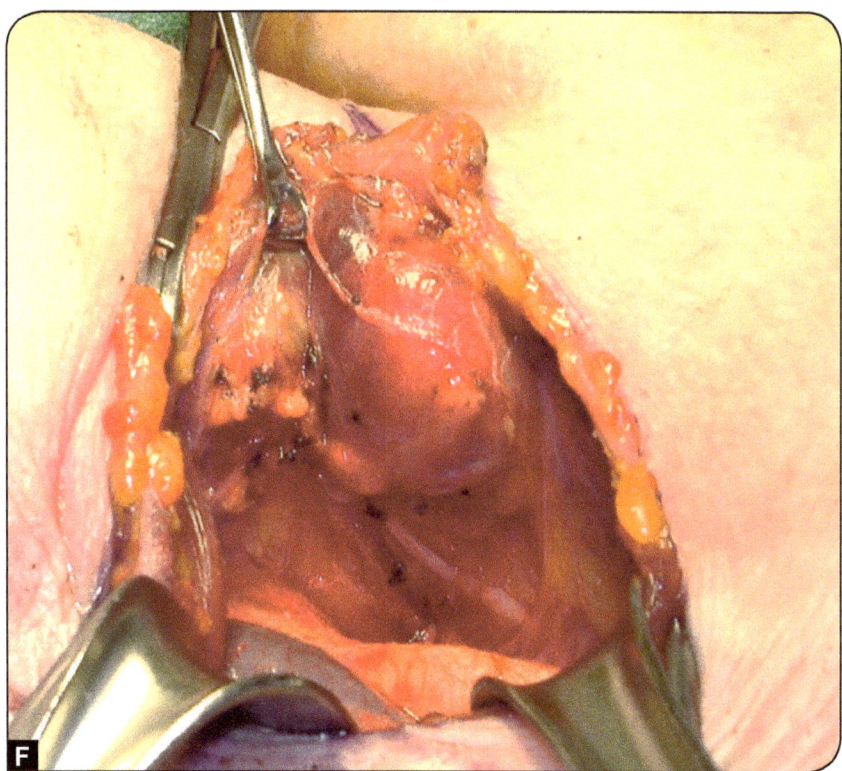

Fig. 1F

- *1G*: Completed pretracheal and right paratracheal dissection. Note that the inferior parathyroid has been preserved (arrow).

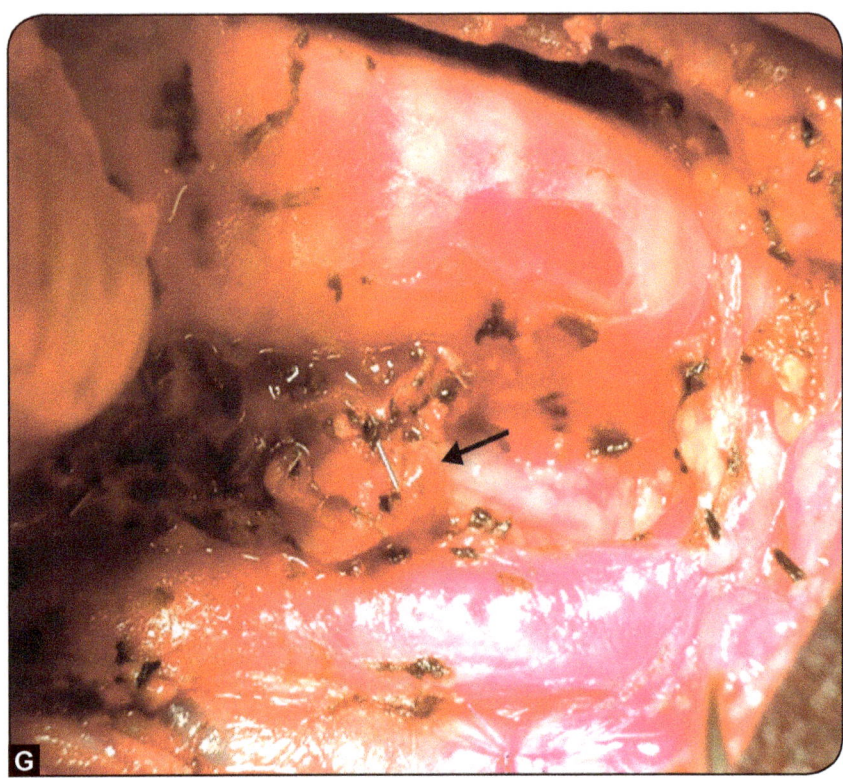

Fig. 1G

With Total Laryngectomy

When a paratracheal and pretracheal node dissection is done in conjunction with a total laryngectomy, the dissection proceeds in the same manner as described in sections 1A to 1G of this chapter.

Steps of dissection with total laryngectomy are as follows:

- *2A*: Once the recurrent laryngeal nerve is identified inferiorly, the nerve is transected.
- *2B*: The paratracheal and pretracheal fatty tissues and lymph nodes are dissected in a superior direction along with the recurrent nerve and the ipsilateral thyroid lobe. In addition, the prelaryngeal (Delphian) lymph node is included. The "block" of dissected tissue is left attached to the larynx at the cricothyroid membrane.

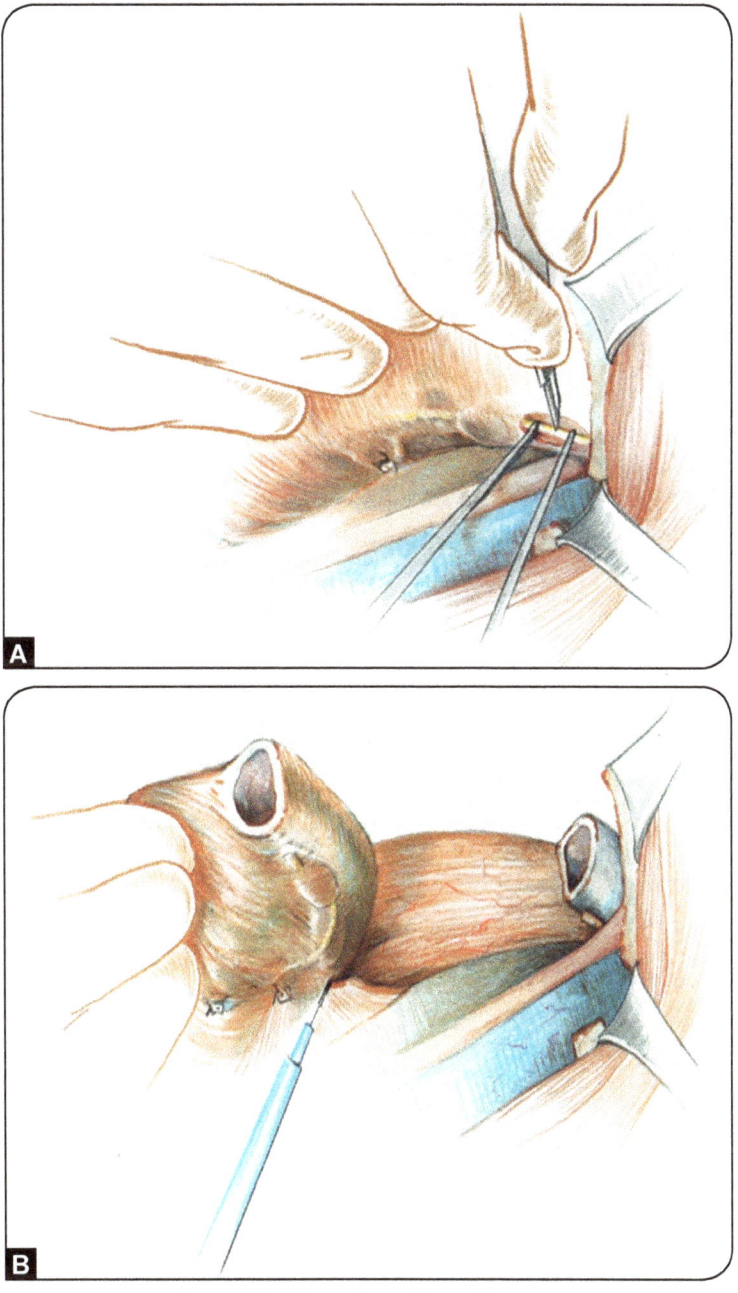

Figs. 2A and B: Dissection with total laryngectomy.

REFERENCES

1. Robbins KT, Shaha AR, Medina JE, et al. Consensus statement on the classification and terminology of neck dissection. Arch Otolaryngol Head Neck Surg. 2008;134(5):536-8.

2. Som PM, Curtin HD, Mancuso AA. Imaging-based nodal classification for evaluation of neck metastatic adenopathy. AJR Am J Roentgenol. 2000;174(3):837-44.

3. Rouviere H. Anatomy of the Human Lymphatic System. Ann Arbor, MI: Edwards Brothers Inc.; 1938.

4. Welsh LW. The normal human laryngeal lymphatics. Ann Otol Rhinol Laryngol. 1964;73:569-82.

5. Johner CH. The lymphatics of the larynx. Otolaryngol Clin North Am. 1970;3(3):439-50.

6. Noguchi S, Noguchi A, Murakami N. Papillary carcinoma of the thyroid. I. Developing pattern of metastasis. Cancer. 1970;26(5):1053-60.

7. Sisson GA, Feldman DE. The management of thyroid carcinoma metastatic to the neck and mediastinum. Otolaryngol Clin North Am. 1980;13(1):119-26.

8. Kelemen PR, Van Herle AJ, Giuliano AE. Sentinel lymphadenectomy in thyroid malignant neoplasms. Arch Surg. 1998;133(3): 288-92.

9. Medina JE, Ferlito A, Robbins KT, et al. Central compartment dissection in laryngeal cancer. Head Neck. 2011;33(5):746-52.

10. Mazzaferri EL, Doherty GM, Steward DL. The pros and cons of prophylactic central compartment lymph node dissection for papillary thyroid carcinoma. Thyroid. 2009;19(7):683-9.

11. Haugen BR, Alexander EK, Bible KC, Doherty GM, Mandel SJ, Nikiforov YE, et al. 2015 American Thyroid Association Management Guidelines for Adult Patients with Thyroid Nodules and Differentiated Thyroid Cancer: The American Thyroid Association Guidelines Task Force on Thyroid Nodules and Differentiated Thyroid Cancer. Thyroid. 2016;26(1):1-133.

12. Wells SA, Asa SL, Dralle H, et al. Revised American Thyroid Association guidelines for the management of medullary thyroid carcinoma: The American Thyroid Association Guidelines Task Force on Medullary Thyroid Carcinoma. Thyroid. 2015;25(6): 567-610.

CHAPTER 11

Retropharyngeal Node Dissection

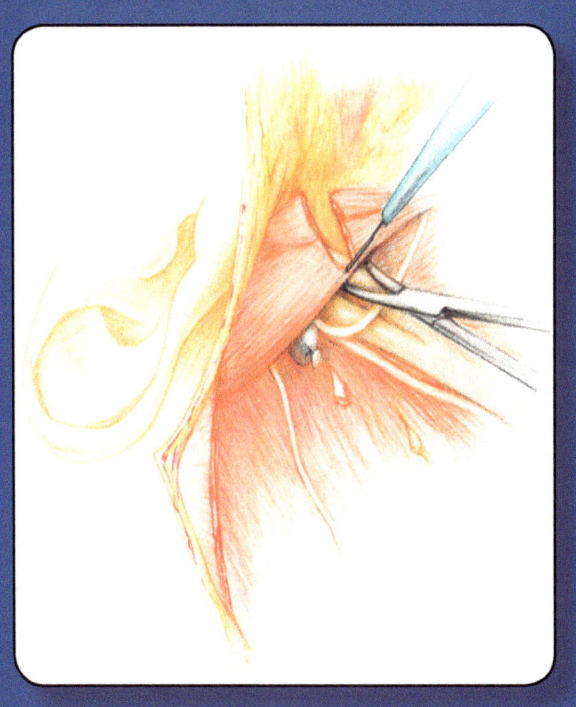
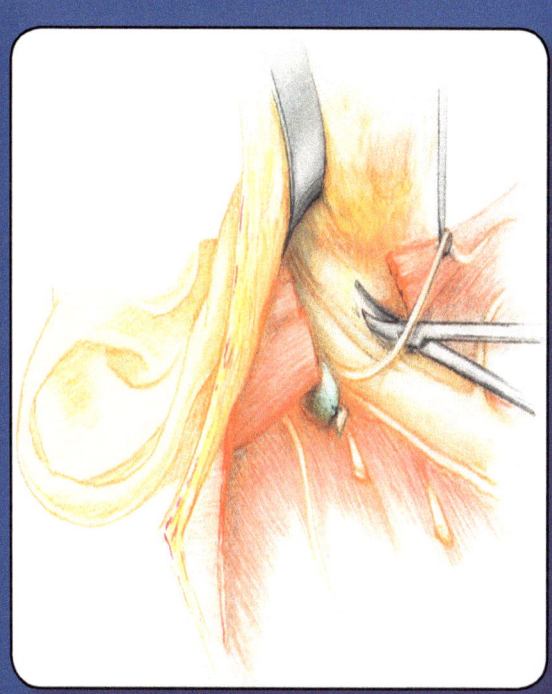

ANATOMY AND CLINICAL RELEVANCE

The retropharyngeal lymph nodes (RPLNs) are located in the retropharyngeal space, within a pad of adipose tissue that extends from about the level of the carotid bifurcation to just inferior to the skull base. This fat pad and lymph nodes are located behind the posterior wall of the pharynx, anterior to the prevertebral fascia and the cervical sympathetic trunk and ganglion, and medial to the internal carotid artery. The RPLNs are divided into medial and lateral groups. The lateral group of nodes, better known as the nodes of Rouvière, are contained within a sliver of adipose tissue located immediately medial to the internal carotid artery (Fig. 1). The number of lateral RPLNs ranges between one and three, and their size varies from 2 to 5 mm. The medial group of nodes lies behind the pharyngeal midline at a level between the first and fourth cervical vertebrae, these lymph nodes are very small and are rarely present in adults.

The RPLNs receive lymphatic drainage from the nasopharynx, tonsil fossa, the walls of the oropharynx and the hypopharynx, and the posterior ethmoid sinuses. Their clinical relevance was first pointed out by Ballantyne[1] in 1964, who found pathologically proven metastases in the RPLNs in 15 of 34 (44%) patients with squamous cell carcinoma of the pharyngeal wall who were treated with total pharyngectomy and dissection of the RPLNs. He also described that involvement of the retropharyngeal nodes by tumor is characteristically signaled by an ipsilateral occipitoparietal headache described by the patient as pain located behind the eye.

Subsequently, in a study designed to assess the frequency of RPLN metastases using enlargement of the RPLN on computed tomography (CT) scans as an indicator of the presence of metastases, McLaughlin et al. found an overall incidence of radiologically "positive" RPLNs of 9% of the patients.[2] The highest incidence was seen in patients with cancer of the nasopharynx (74%) and the pharyngeal walls (19%). They also noted that in patients with advanced cancer of the walls of the oropharynx and hypopharynx, the incidence of radiologically positive RPLNs was higher in patients with cervical metastases (N+ necks) than in those with an N0 neck (pharyngeal wall: N+ 21%, N0 16%; hypopharynx: N+ 9%, N0 0%). Others have reported similar findings.[3]

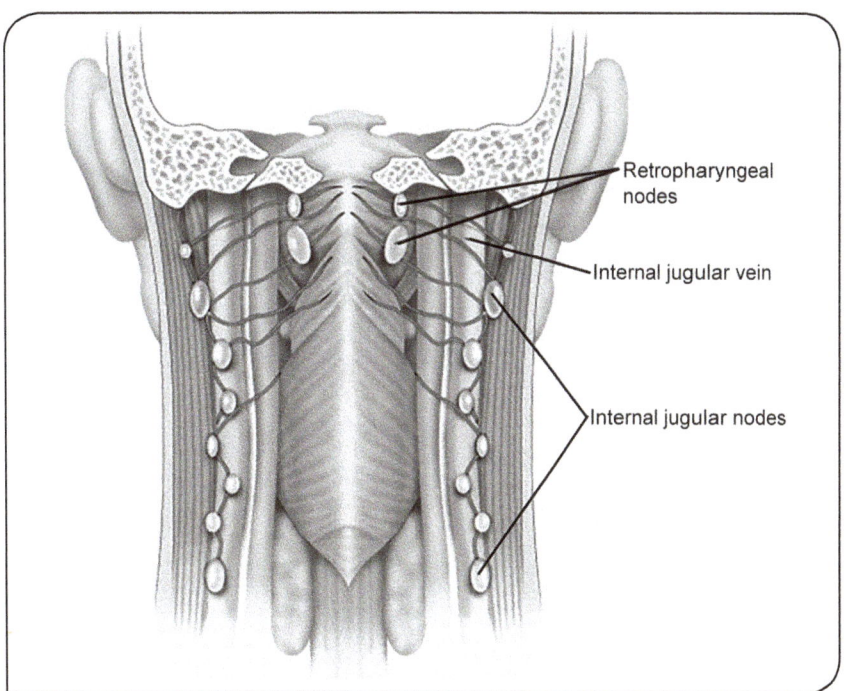

Fig. 1: Anatomy of the retropharyngeal lymph nodes.
Source: Reprinted with permission from Vasan NR, Medina JE. Retropharyngeal lymph nodes.
Oper Tech Otolaryngol Head Neck Surg. 2004;15(3):180-3.

In the current era of chemoradiation for the management of squamous cell carcinomas of the oropharynx and hypopharynx, the retropharyngeal nodes are treated electively with radiation, in patients with obvious metastases in the neck. Likewise, obviously positive RPLNs are initially treated with chemoradiation. However, today, an increasing number of selected patients with squamous cell carcinoma of the oropharynx are being treated with transoral robotic surgery and neck dissection, with the intent of managing the disease with surgery as the single treatment modality. As a result, the clinician must decide when to remove the RPLNs. Moore et al.[4] have provided useful information for this decision-making process in patients with cancer of the tonsil. They found that 9% of patients with tumors staged T1–T2 and 57 % of patients with T3–T4 tumors had RPLN metastases. On the other hand, none of the patients whose neck was staged N0–N2b had RPLN metastases, while 25.8% of the patients with more advanced neck disease had them.

Until similar information is available for tumors of the oropharyngeal walls and the hypopharynx, dissection of the RPLN should be considered if the intent is to treat the patient with transoral robotic surgery and neck dissection, alone.

INDICATIONS

A retropharyneal lymph node dissection is indicated in the treatment of tumors of the tonsillar fossa, oropharyngeal and hypopharyngeal walls:

- When the primary tumor is treated with surgery, transorally or otherwise, and the CT or positron emission tomography (PET)/CT show findings suggestive of metastasis in the RPLNs.
- When the primary tumor is treated with surgery, transorally or otherwise, the CT and/or PET/CT show no findings suggestive of metastases in the RPLNs and the intention is to treat the patients with surgery alone. Removal and histopathological examination of the RPLNs provides information necessary to determine if adjuvant postoperative treatment with radiation, with or with concomitant chemotherapy is indicated.
- When performing salvage surgery for tumors of the oropharynx and hypopharynx previously treated with radiation with or without chemotherapy.
- Occasionally, to remove metastases from papillary thyroid cancer. Interestingly, unlike squamous cell carcinoma, metastases from papillary thyroid carcinoma tend to grow slowly in a pushing rather than infiltrating manner. Consequently, they may not invade the carotid or the prevertebral fascia, even when they are several centimeters in diameter, and can be removed with relative ease.

SURGICAL TECHNIQUE

Dissection of the retropharyngeal nodes can be performed separately or in continuity with the resection of the primary tumor. When it is done electively, this operation is relatively simple and it takes only a few minutes. On the other hand, when the RPLNs are grossly involved by tumor, the operation may be difficult and sometimes not feasible. The proximity of the nodes to the internal carotid artery and prevertebral structures is such that these structures may be involved as soon as tumor extends beyond the capsule of the lymph nodes.

- *2A*: Following completion of the neck dissection, the posterior belly of digastric and the hypoglossal nerve should be clearly visible. Using a Sewell or a Deaver retractor, placed between the carotid artery laterally and the pharynx medially, these structures are retracted superiorly. Alternatively, the posterior belly of digastric and the styloid muscles are divided to facilitate the dissection. Identification and dissection of the retropharyngeal space is much easier after a laryngopharyngectomy as the retropharyngeal space has already been identified and the removal of the larynx facilitates retraction of the suprahyoid musculature.

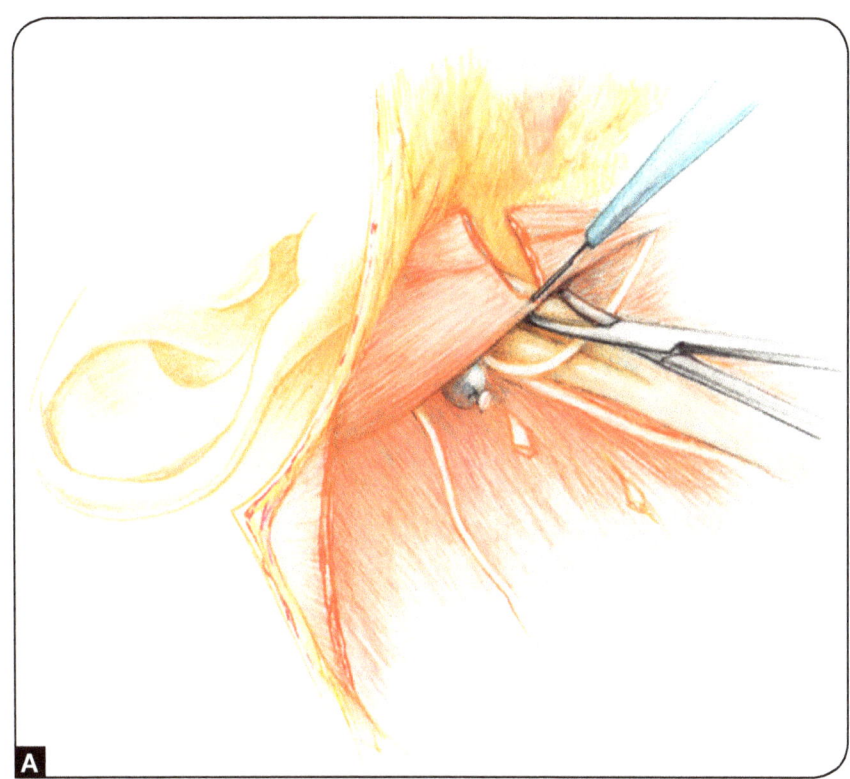

Fig. 2A

- *2B*: The anterior most layer of the prevertebral fascia is incised at a point immediately medial to the carotid bifurcation.

- *2C*: The retropharyngeal fat pad is then identified and dissected from below, upwards, using either tenotomy scissors or electrocautery. The latter should be used with caution to avoid damaging the cervical sympathetic trunk, which is located posterior and somewhat lateral to the fat pad.

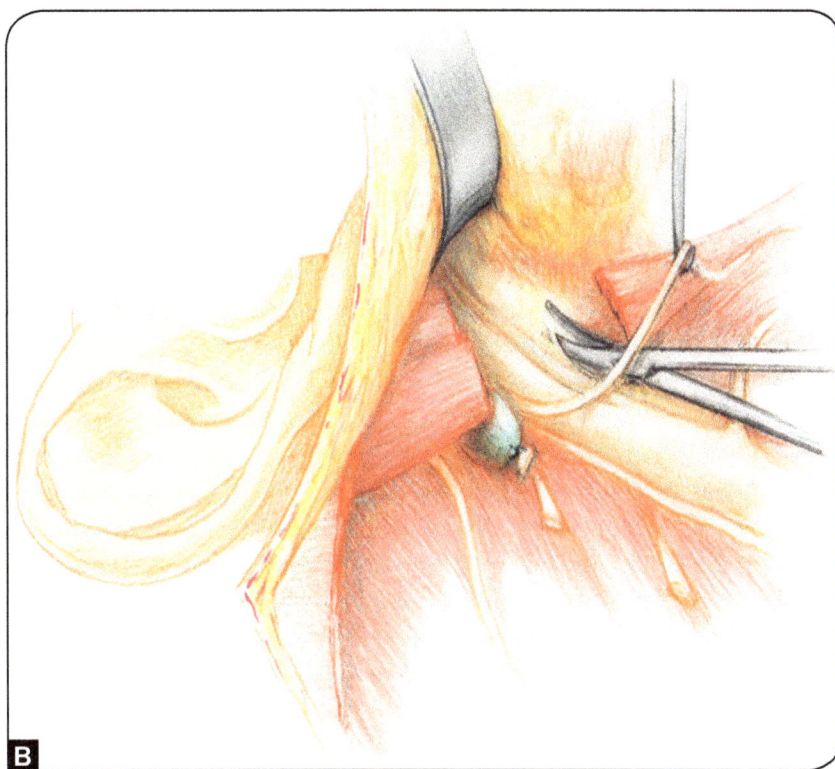

Fig. 2B

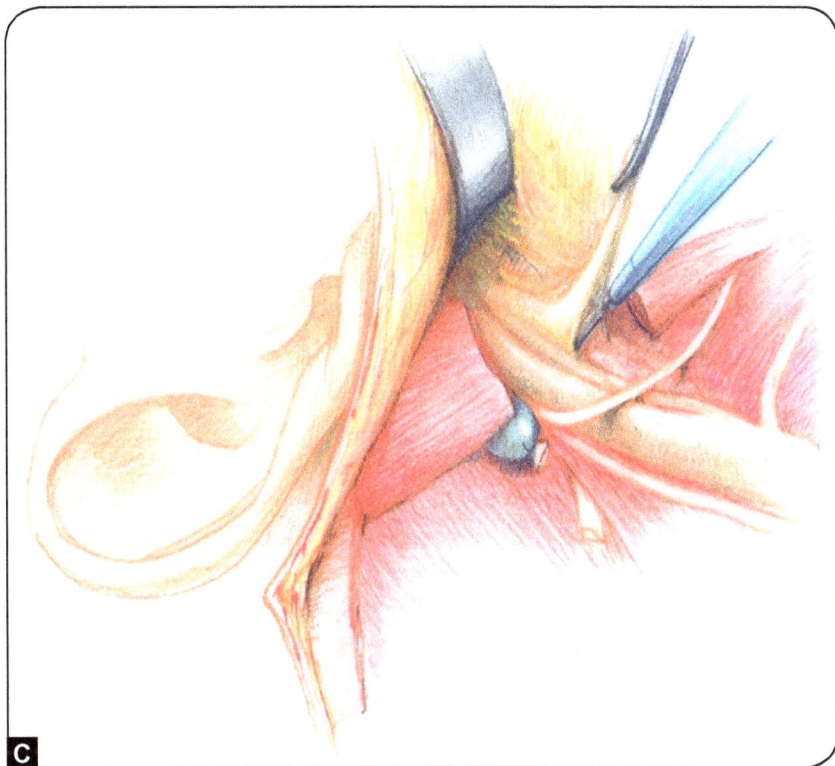

Fig. 2C

- *2D*: The dissection of this fat pad is continued in a cephalad direction. In doing this, the cervical sympathetic ganglion can be easily mistaken for an enlarged retropharyngeal node, thus, it is preferable to identify it and keep it under vision. Likewise, to avoid inadvertent injury to the internal carotid artery, it is best to be constantly aware of its location or to have it under direct vision. If the dissection is carried in the right plane, it is usually bloodless with the exception of few parapharyngeal veins. These are controlled with either ties or bipolar diathermy. Due to the close proximity of the sympathetic trunk, monopolar cautery should be used with caution if at all. It is also preferable to avoid ligaclips because they can produce artifact that interfere with future imaging studies of the area. The final cut, below the base of the skull, is done with scissors and the specimen is delivered.

- *2E*: The completed dissection is shown here.

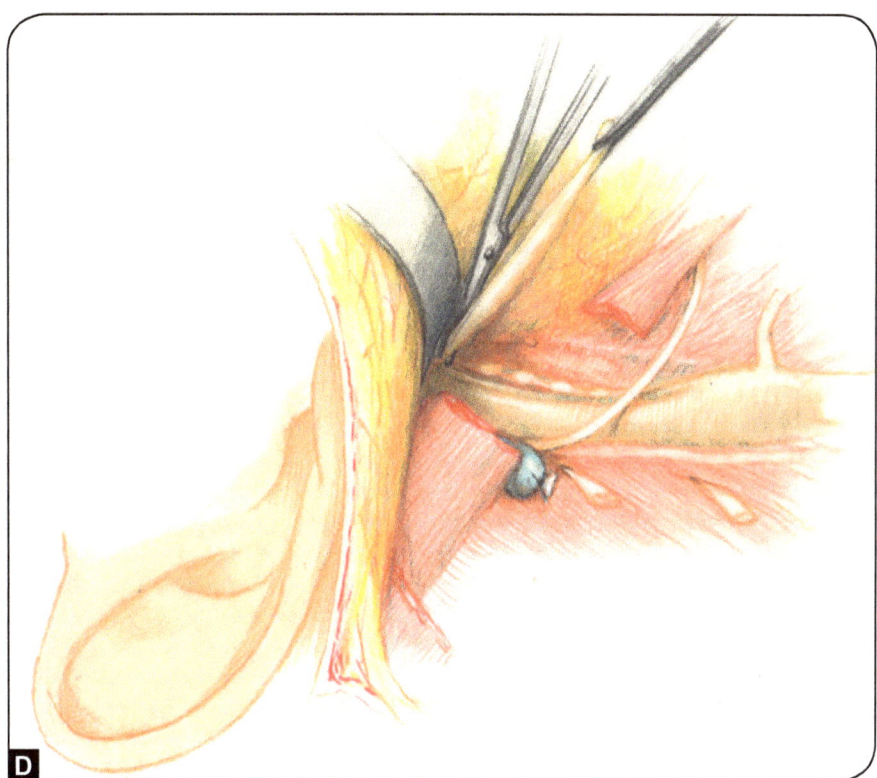

Fig. 2D

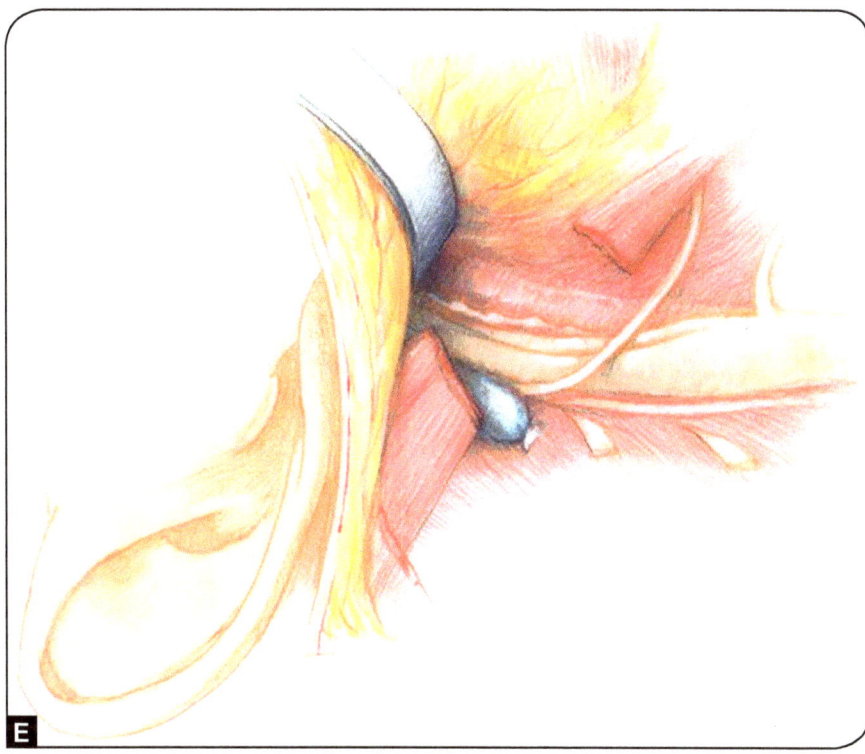

Fig. 2E

REFERENCES

1. Ballantyne AJ. Significance of retropharyngeal nodes in cancer of the head and neck. Am J Surg. 1964;108:500-4.
2. McLaughlin MP, Mendenhall WM, Mancuso AA, et al. Retropharyngeal adenopathy as a predictor of outcome in squamous cell carcinoma of the head and neck. Head Neck. 1995;17(3):190-8.
3. Amatsu M, Mohri M, Kinishi M. Significance of retropharyngeal node dissection at radical surgery for carcinoma of the hypo-pharynx and cervical esophagus. Laryngoscope. 2001;111(6):1099-103.
4. Moore EJ, Ebrahimi A, Price DL, et al. Retropharyngeal lymph node dissection in oropharyngeal cancer treated with transoral robotic surgery. Laryngoscope. 2013;123(7):1676-81.

Index

Note: Page numbers followed by *f* refer to figure.